GASTROSTOMY

Edited by **Pavel Kohout**

Gastrostomy
Edited by Pavel Kohout

Published by InTech
Janeza Trdine 9, 51000 Rijeka, Croatia

Publishing Process Manager Silvia Vlase

Technical Editor Teodora Smiljanic

Cover Designer InTech Design Team

Additional hard copies can be obtained from orders@intechopen.com

Gastrostomy, Edited by Pavel Kohout
p. cm.
ISBN 978-953-307-365-1

For EU product safety concerns:
IN TECH d.o.o., Prolaz Marije Krucifikse Kozulić 3, 51000 Rijeka, Croatia,
info@intechopen.com or visit our website at intechopen.com.

Meet the editor

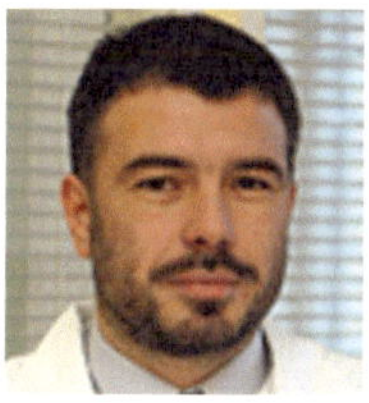

Dr Pavel Kohout graduated from the Medical Faculty at Charles University in Prague in 1986. His research interests include gastroenterology (especially inflammatory bowel diseases, coeliac disease and acute pancreatitis), intensive metabolic care and nutrition (including home parenteral and enteral nutrition, percutaneous endoscopic gastrostomy and standards of nutrition care in hospitals). He is currently Head of the Center of nutrition and Nutrition team in Teaching Thomayer's Hospital Prague (Czech Republic) and Head of Metabolic ICU. Dr Kohout is also a member of: Executive committee of Czech Society for Clinical Nutrition and Intensive Metabolic Care, Executive committee of Czech Society of Nutrition and a member of Czech as well as European gastroenterology and nutrition societies. He has authored 4 monographs in Czech language (Percutaneous Endoscopic Gastrostomy, Basics of Clinical Nutrition, Chapters from Clinical Nutrition, Non-invasive Diagnostic of Small bowel), and about 120 original and review papers in international journals. During his career he has introduced more than 1500 percutaneous endoscopic gastrostomies into patients from 6 weeks to 98 years of age.

Contents

Preface XI

Part 1 Gastrostomy in Children 1

Chapter 1 **Advances in Gastrostomy Placement and Care in Children 3**
Stephen Adams and Anies Mahomed

Chapter 2 **Gastrostomy in Pediatric Patients 17**
Brian W. Gray, Ana Ruzic and George B. Mychaliska

Chapter 3 **Percutaneous Endoscopic Gastrostomy in Pediatric Patients 25**
Omar I. Saadah

Part 2 Indications of Gastrostomy in the Adults 49

Chapter 4 **Percutaneous Endoscopic Gastrostomy in Neurological Patients 51**
David T. Burke and Andrew I. Geller

Chapter 5 **Defining the Indications for Prophylactic Percutaneous Endoscopic Gastrostomy Tubes in Surgically Treated Head and Neck Cancer Patients 73**
Jason Foster, Peter Filocamo, William Brady, Thom Loree and John F. Gibbs

Part 3 Gastrostomy Techniques 81

Chapter 6 **The Place of Laparoscopic Gastrostomy in the Surgical Armamentarium 83**
Philip Ng Cheng Hin

Chapter 7 **Video-Assisted Gastrostomy in Children 91**
Torbjörn Backman, Malin Mellberg, Helén Sjöwie, Magnus Anderberg and Einar Arnbjörnsson

Chapter 8 **The Twin-Stoma Gastrostomy and the LOOPPEG® 3G Tube 119**
Ah San, Pang

Part 4 Complications of Gastrostomy 129

Chapter 9 **High Level of Intra-Gastric Pressure is Risk Factor for Patients with Percutaneous Endoscopic Gastrostomy (PEG) 131**
Michiaki Kudo, Nobuyuki Kanai, Toshiaki Hirasawa, Takayuki Asao and Hiroyuki Kuwano

Part 5 Psychosomatic Aspects of Gastrostomy 139

Chapter 10 **Psychosomatic Manifestations of Gastrostomy in Head and Neck Surgery 141**
Francisco Hernández Altemir, Sofía Hernández Montero, Susana Hernández Montero, Elena Hernández Montero and Manuel Moros Peña

Preface

Life is an interesting possibility to realize a dream.
Paolo Coelho, *The Alchemist*

The gastrostomy placement is a method of providing nutrition to the patients who are unable to eat. The possibility of feeding the patients, who were unable to eat, has been physicians' dream for a long time.

The first way was a surgical introduction using open laparotomy in malignant patients, which was used since the 19th century. In the 20th century radiological, and later (since the 80s) endoscopic techniques, were implemented and the number of patients and new indications was increased. Gastrostomy became the standard procedure in patients with various causes of feeding disturbances from birth to the advanced age, and by the end of the 20th century, Percutaneous Endoscopic Gastrostomy (PEG) served as a gold standard.

At this time the most frequent groups for gastrostomy introduction are children with various disturbances, geriatric patients (especially with cerebral stroke and demency), patients with neurological impairment and mostly patients with malignancies. Home enteral nutrition is suitable for all these groups of patients and it is more easy with gastronomy, so probably this is the dream for patients – to be at home with realtives and loved ones despite of their troubles.

It is no wonder that the individual chapters are focused on children, neurological patients and the patients, who most benefit from the introduction of gastrostomy, namely head and neck cancer patients.

The new indications (especially in very young children) required new techniques such as: laparoscopic gastrostomy, laparoscopy assisted endoscopic gastrostomy with/without fundoplication, ultrasonography assisted gastronomy etc.

This is the reason, why you can find in this book the chapters about new techniques of gastrostomy introduction - video-laparoscopy techniques, twin gastrostomy and other.

I realized my dream too, during last 18 years, our team introduced more than 2000 percutaneous endoscopical gastrostomies (about 140 in children below 15 years) from children 6 weeks old to a female-patient 98 years old (she lived about 3 years longer with total enteral nutrition and with full mobility), more than 50 introduction of gastrostomies contraindicated in the other endoscopy rooms. Therefore, we have become the learning center for PEG introduction and the medical center, which solves the complicated cases for the whole Czech Republic.

I was very proud that I got the opportunity to be present at the birth of a new book about gastrostomy.

This book does not serve as a basic textbook, but as an interesting reading material and as an aid for physicians who are already familiar with the indication for gastrostomy and want to know more.

Prague 28th October 2011

Pavel Kohout
IInd Dept of Internal Diseases
Thomayer´s Hospital,
Prague,
Czech Republic

Part 1

Gastrostomy in Children

1

Advances in Gastrostomy Placement and Care in Children

Stephen Adams and Anies Mahomed
Royal Alexandra Children's Hospital, Brighton
United Kingdom

1. Introduction

Gastrostomy Placement in Children has advanced much in recent years. We have experience in standard techniques of open and percutaneous endoscopic Gastrostomy placement and continue to expand our surgical portfolio to include minimally invasive techniques for gastrostomy placement. Over the past 2 years our department has placed 49 new gastrostomy devices, (Age: Median 2.6 years, Range 0-18) for a wide range of diagnoses.
In this chapter we chart the history of the Gastrostomy in children, indications and methods for placement including an overview of more recent techniques, their risks and benefits.

2. Historical perspective

Gastrostomy is probably the first operation performed on the human stomach and was successfully practised in adults from the mid to late 1800s. The credit for being the first surgeon to describe and successfully establish a gastostomy in a human belongs to Sédillot of Strasbourg. He published his article "De Ia Gastrostomie Fistuleuse" in France in 1846. The main initial complication of the procedure was development of peritonitis in the immediate post-operative phase. This was ameliorated somewhat by development of the technique to involve suturing a portion of the stomach to the peritoneum and leaving several days prior to opening the presenting area of the stomach. In these pre-Listerian days success was significantly limited and no patients were recorded as surviving until 1876. This is likely to have been affected by the underlying (usually malignant) conditions for which the procedure was being used.
Further developments were aimed at preventing leak and related skin excoriation. Notable amongst the earlier success were two French surgeons named Fontan and Pénières who in the late 1800s described a new technique whereby all the layers of the stomach were used in the creation of a type of valve. A Belgian surgeon named Dépage also described the use of a mucous lined tube in the creation of the fistula. By 1899 a Japanese surgeon named Watsudjii had published a modification of these techniques such as to bring the gastrostomy to the skin through the rectus abdominus muscle, thus creating the first continent gastrostomy. Subsequent descriptions and modifications of what we now recognise as an open gastrostomy were made by many and names such as Janeway, Spivack and Stamm will come to mind when one considers this history further. (Cunha 1946)

The next significant change in technique came in 1980 when Gauderer and Ponsky first described a method for Gastrostomy placement which avoided the previously associated laparotomy. The Percutaneous Endoscopic Gastrostomy (PEG) was described in a cohort of high risk patients, around one third of whom were children. The technique which will be explored in more detail later in this chapter was to revolutionise our concept of gastrostomy placement. (Gauderer et al. 1980)

The first uses of Gastrostomy in children were for treating patients with caustic oesophageal strictures. Subsequently the incidence of such strictures has markedly reduced and the indication for gastrostomy has changed. Its use in neonates, which was more prevalent in the 1970s and 1980s, has now reduced as neonatal and peri-operative care has improved. The population of neuro-developmentally delayed children has increased dramatically as the capacity to provide advanced neonatal care has developed. This group now presents the most common requirement for gastrostomy placement in current paediatric practice. (Gauderer 1992)

3. Indications and assessment for gastrostomy placement

The three main indications for gastrostomy placement in children are;

1. Long term feeding
2. Gastric decompression
3. A combination of the above

Additional uses include the administration of medication, gastric access for passage of oesophageal dilators and gastroscopy. (Gauderer 1992)

The European Society for Clinical Nutrition and Metabolism (ESPEN) has issued a consensus statement which provides guidelines in relation to Percutaneous Endoscopic Gastrostomy (Lo et al. 2005). These suggest that when oral feeding is no longer possible or adequate for an expected duration of greater than 2-3 weeks there is an indication for PEG placement. Additionally these guidelines suggest that a jejunal extension of the PEG tube be placed when there is a significant risk of aspiration. The placement of any form of adjuvant device for feeding requires careful consideration and planning and whilst the ESPEN statement does provide guidance, the authors feel that they should not be regarded as rules to follow, indeed many surgeons will not consider placing a surgical gastrostomy unless it will be required for 3 months or more. (Georgeson 1997)

Given that the most common group to present to the paediatric surgeon for consideration of Gastrostomy placement is the neurologically compromised child it is prudent to consider the issues of Gastro-Oesophageal Reflux (GOR) and upper GI dysmotility prior to proceeding. A combined anti-reflux procedure and Gastrostomy placement can be well advised in a proven case of GOR, since placement of Gastrostomy alone is known to potentially worsen the GOR. (Chung & Georgeson 1998). The main indications for Gastrostomy are listed in Table 1.

Assessment of the child presenting for Gastrostomy placement should commence with a comprehensive clinical history, taking particular note of Acute Life-Threatening Events (ALTEs) and progressive neurological disease likely to mandate an anti-reflux procedure in the future. Diagnostic imaging should involve an upper gastro-intestinal (GI) contrast study in the first instance, this provides both anatomical and functional information likely to influence decision making. In the absence of a clinical history to suggest GOR it may seem reasonable to base the decision making on this evaluation alone, however a contrast study which does not demonstrate reflux certainly does not exclude it. There are several other investigations in the clinician's armamentarium to help in making this diagnosis.

Indication	Underlying Disease
Inability to swallow	Neurological Disorders (>50% all patients)
	Multiple Congenital Malformations
	Oropharyngeal dymotility
	Epidermolysis Bullosa
	Others
Inadequate Calorific Intake	Cystic Fibrosis
	Congenital Heart Disease
	Chronic Respiratory Failure
	Chemotherapy in oncologic disease
	Others
Special Feeding Requirements	Unpalatable formula in multiple food allergies
	Unpalatable formula or reliable Gastric access in metabolic diseases
	Unpalatable medications in renal failure
Continuous Enteral Feeding	Short Bowel Syndrome
	Malabsorption

Table 1. Indications and underlying diseases in paediatric patients requiring a PEG - adapted from Frohlich et al (2010)

Twenty-four hour Oesophageal pH monitoring is considered the gold standard test for establishing a diagnosis of GOR. A pH probe is placed just above the lower oesophageal sphincter and recordings are made on a portable device for the ensuing day and night. Gastric-emptying can be assessed to a degree on an Upper GI contrast study, but quantification of emptying can only be made using a Nuclear Medicine "Milk Scan". The presence of significantly delayed gastric emptying may be an indication for a gastric outlet procedure possibly in addition to fundoplication and gastrostomy. Oesophageal manometry and oesophagoscopy, with biopsy, if required can prove a useful adjunct in complex clinical scenarios. (Chung & Georgeson 1998)

4. Standard technique for PEG placement

The most widely accepted modern technique for paediatric Gastrostomy placement is the Percutaneous Endoscopic Gastrostomy (PEG) as first described by Gauderer and Ponsky in 1980. This technique achieves a sutureless apposition of the stomach to the anterior abdominal wall with a tube Gastrostomy being left in-situ. It was first described with equipment that was presently available, now there are many specialised kits available from multiple manufacturers to achieve a similar outcome. The basic premise is summarised in Figure 1.

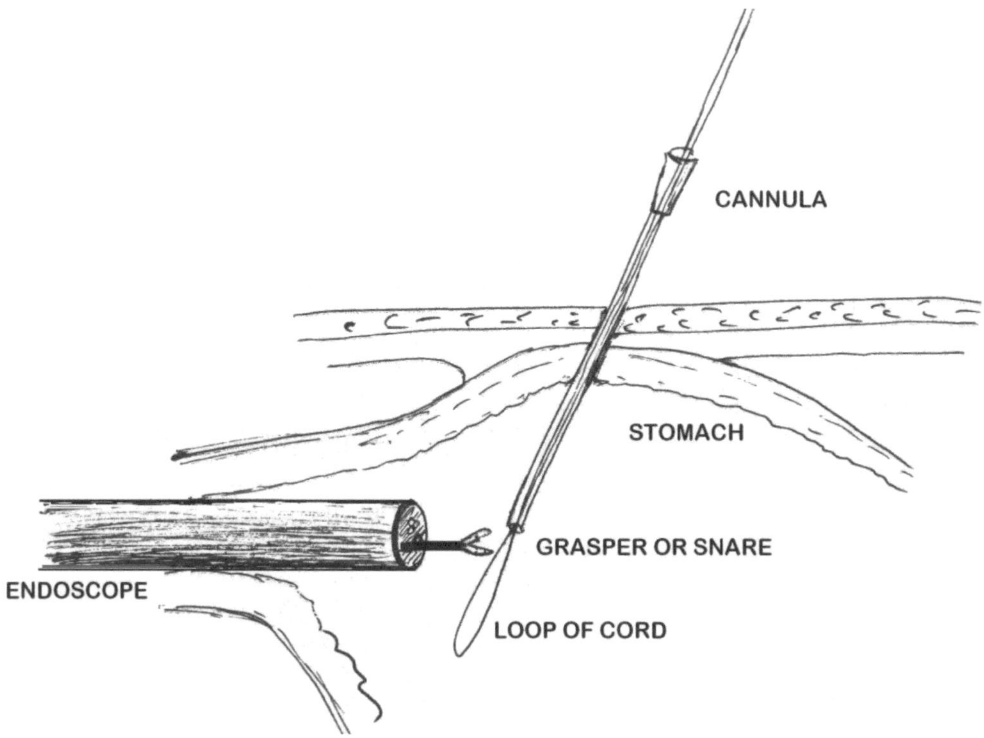

Fig. 1. Depiction of PEG placement – adapted from (Gauderer, Ponsky, & Izant, 1980, Fig 3)

The stomach is intubated with a flexible endoscope which has a working channel. It is insufflated with air in order to try to push the colon, liver and spleen away from the proposed gastrostomy site. A cannula is placed via the anterior abdominal wall into the stomach under endoscopic vision. A thread passed via the cannula is grasped by the endoscopist and withdrawn through the mouth. A catheter is attached to the string which is then used to pull the catheter down the oesophagus and out through the Gastrostomy site, the catheter is shaped such that the presenting portion is narrow but widens to the full catheter diameter and an internal flange resides against the anterior wall of stomach. A flange at skin level enables maintenance of apposition between the stomach and anterior abdominal wall.

The initial concern with this technique was the potential to pierce the colon and this is in fact a well documented risk, in a recent selection of paediatric case series the rate of this complication is 1 - 2%. The risk of the same complication when the gastrostomy is created in the traditional manner is probably minute and is rarely reported. (Cook 1969) The overall complication rate of standard PEG insertion is variously reported as between 5 and 17%. The major complications are summarised in Table 2 which is adapted from a single centre study of 448 standard paediatric PEG insertions.

Major Complications	%
Death (30 days post-PEG)	1.1
Procedure-related	0.2 (1/448 due to PEG related sepsis)
Oesophageal Perforation	0.2
Peritonitis	1.6
Gastrocolic fistula	1.1
Intra-abdominal bleeding	0.7
Necrosis (PEG Migration)	0.4
Major infection	0.9
GOR after PEG (new or more)	2.9
Major granulation tissue	1.8
Buried bumper	2.5
Miscellaneous (Mainly needle perforations of colon and stomach)	3.3
Total	*16.7*

Table 2. Major Complications of PEG insertion, adapted from (Vervloessem et al. 2009)

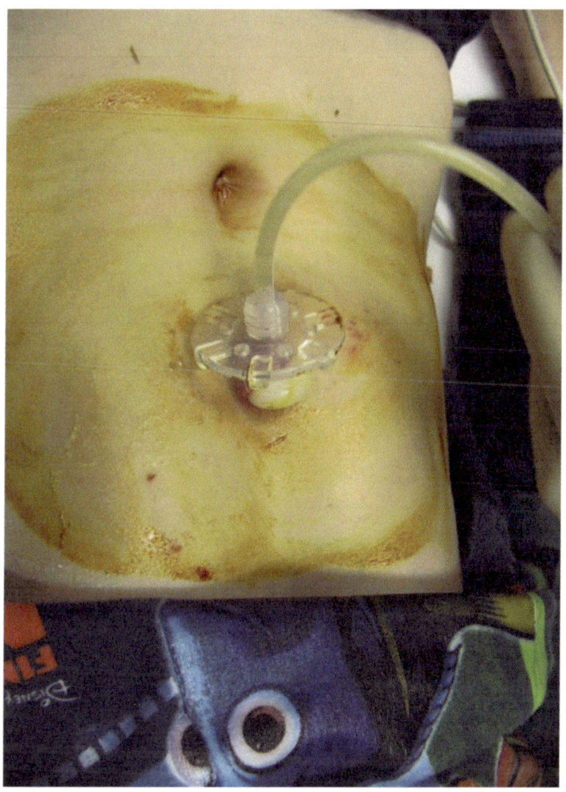

Fig. 2. Complication: extrusion of a Corflo® gastrostomy device

Common, but more minor, complications include minimal granulation tissue, tube migration, dislodgement (this can be a major complication if it occurs within the first 4-6 weeks), stomal enlargement, leakage, skin irritation/breakdown and tube blockage. The gastrostomy tube may be an annoyance to the child and some children with PEG avoid spending time prone, this may lead to developmental issues with upper torso and head control. When it is no longer required the Gastrostomy tube is removed and the stoma permitted to close. The stoma usually closes rapidly however occasionally this can take several weeks and be problematic due to profuse leakage of gastric content. Rarely a persistent gastro-cutaneous fistula will require surgical closure. (Borkowski 1998)
Contra-indications to traditional PEG placement are rarely absolute. Extreme kypho-scoliosis, previous upper GI surgery, hepato- or spleno-megaly, colonic interposition, presence of ventriculo-peritoneal shunt and Situs Inversus should all be considered to present significantly increased risk during PEG placement. In this scenario it is wise to consider whether additional measures should be taken for intra-operative imaging of at-risk structures. This can be achieved with laparoscopy or additional radiographical imaging at the time of PEG placement. Such techniques are discussed later in this chapter.

5. Gastrostomy devices

The Malecot, dePezzer and Foley catheters are examples of tubes used when creating an open gastrostomy. More recently specific gastrostomy balloon catheters have been produced. The type of Gastrostomy tube used in placing a PEG usually has a plastic internal disc, examples include the CorFlo® and Freka® PEG tubes (see figure 3).

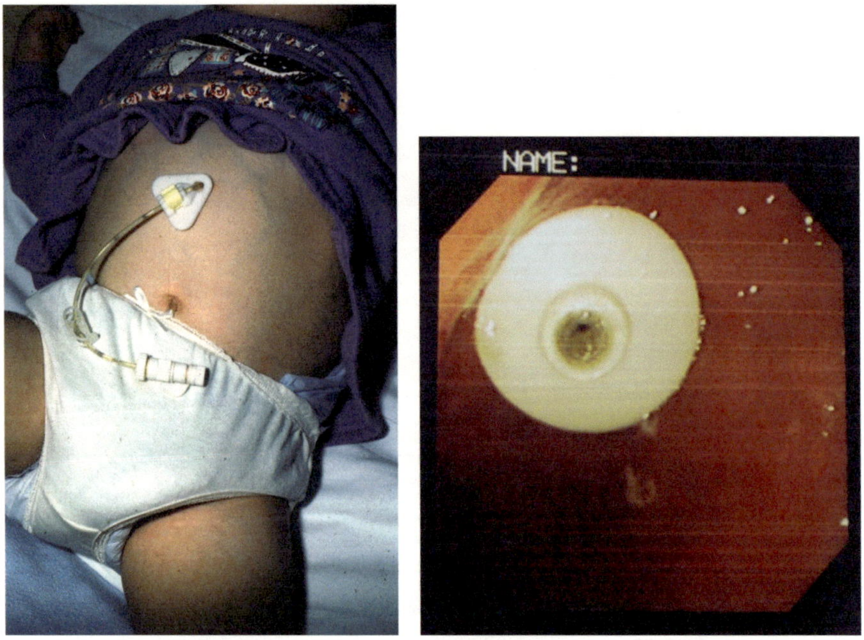

(a) (b)

Fig. 3. FREKA® gastrostomy device – (a) External view and (b) endoscopic view demonstrating disc secured against anterior gastric wall

Button Gastrostomy devices (Figures 4 and 5) have emerged onto the market in the past number of years. They have a much lower profile to the patient's abdomen as there is no requirement for tubing to be connected at all times. Instead, the feed tubing is attached, usually via insertion of a plastic nipple into a valve on the button, only at times when feeding is required. The majority of buttons currently in use have a balloon internally holding them in the stomach. There are buttons however available with an internal plastic cage, these are felt by some surgeons to be more difficult to pull out by accident and may thus be more suitable for some patients.

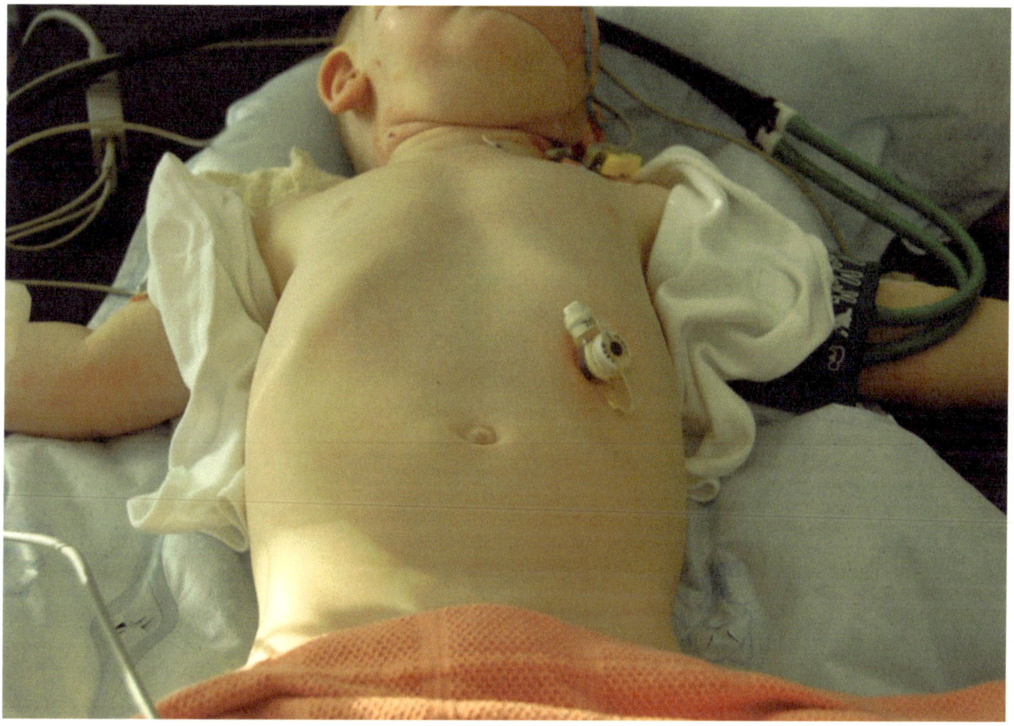

Fig. 4. Infant with button balloon gastrostomy device in situ

A variety of other specialised devices have been produced which enable radiological placement of a gastrostomy tube and also devices to access the jejunum via a gastrostomy, either as an extension to a gastrostomy device or as an exclusive gastro-jejunal tube.

The utility of these jejunal tubes as a long-term solution for enteral feeding, particularly for a child with severe gastro-oesophageal reflux, is debatable due to the high rate of associated morbidity and in particular the frequency of tube displacement. In one reported series of 14 patients with gastro-jejunal tubes there were 65 complications reported in 18 tube insertions (4.6 complications per child). The most common problem was tube migration/displacement (43 episodes). (Godbole et al. 2002)

The other disadvantage of jejunal feeding is the inability to bolus feed and thus feeds must be given continuously over at least 14 hours. These tubes can provide a stop-gap for enteral nutrition when necessary and there is supportive evidence for the nutritional benefits, however they will not usually be the best choice for ongoing nutrition.

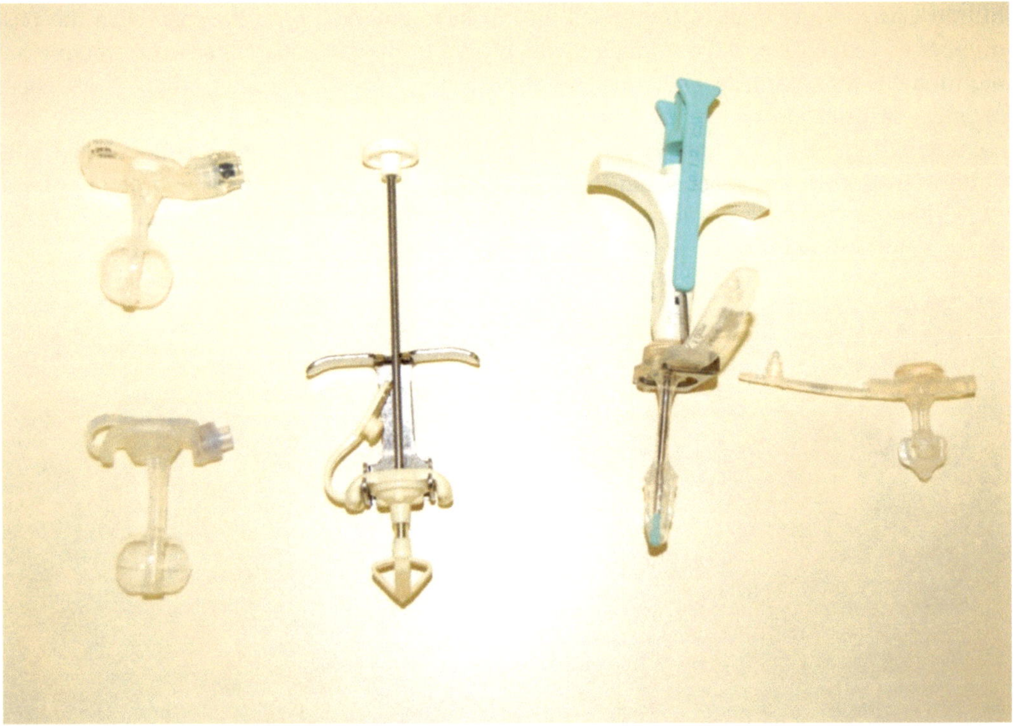

Fig. 5. A Selection of balloon and cage type button gastrostomy devices and their deployment/removal tools

The development of buttons and their better acceptance by parents has led to the development of techniques by which a button gastrostomy can be placed at the initial operation. This technique is addressed in detail in the next section. If this technique is not utilised, many surgeons will replace an initial PEG tube with a button only under a second anaesthetic, usually when the gastrostomy tract has matured and several months post initial PEG placement.

6. Changes in techniques for gastrostomy placement

Aside from the sea-change already described following the introduction of the PEG technique in 1979, there have been major developments in the area of minimal access surgery and interventional radiology. Here we discuss the methods and potential benefits of minimal access surgery and interventional radiology in the placement of gastrostomy devices.

6.1 Solely laparoscopic technique

Laparoscopy has developed a significant role in paediatric surgery, it is used widely for fundoplication of the stomach and many other operations that previously required a more invasive approach (Chung & Georgeson 1998). The visualisation of structures neighbouring the stomach when a laparoscope is used is felt by many to ameliorate the risks of collateral injury associated with PEG placement.

The purely laparoscopic technique was described initially in a porcine model and then utilised in children (G. Stringel et al. 1993). It requires placement of 1 laparoscopic camera and 2 working ports in an anaesthetised patient. The stomach is visualised and brought near to the anterior abdominal wall. A needle is introduced and seen to pass into the lesser curve of the stomach, apparently confirmed by a rush of air through the needle. The stomach is secured to the anterior abdominal wall with a T-fastener. A wire is then passed into the stomach and a series of dilators are used until the stoma is large enough to accept the gastrostomy tube. The system is tested by passing water into the stomach via NG tube and then aspirating it via the new gastrostomy.
The element of uncertainty remains in regard to intra-luminal placement of the gastrostomy with this method, hence the test with water as described, and the same authors also describe a similar technique for laparoscopic assisted placement.

6.2 Laparoscopic-assisted PEG +/- Laparoscopic fundoplication

This technique follows the original principles of PEG placement (Gauderer et al. 1980) with the addition of concurrent laparoscopic visualisation of the abdominal viscera. This enables avoidance of injury to neighbouring viscera and the other reported benefit is that PEG placement can be achieved specifically into the lesser curvature of the stomach which has been seen by some to decrease the risk of developing gastro-oesophageal reflux subsequent to PEG placement, this is of particular relevance in neuro-developmentally delayed children (B. G. Stringel et al. 1995).

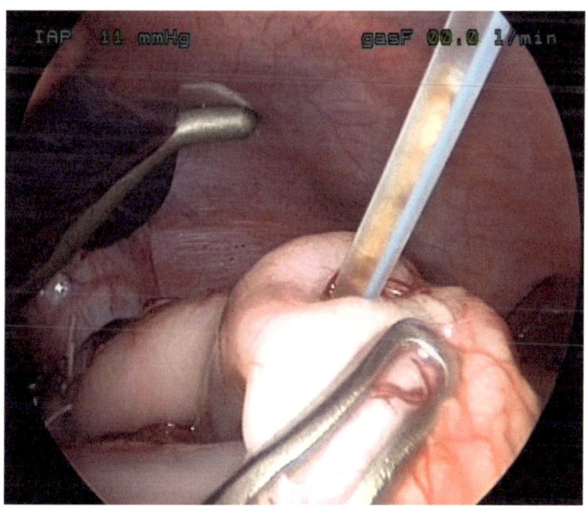

Fig. 6. Clear views obtained during Laparoscopic assisted FREKA® gastrostomy placement in a patient undergoing a fundoplication

This technique is performed by undertaking laparoscopy with a camera port in the umbilicus (5mm or 10mm) and a 5mm working port placed under vision in the upper abdomen or epigastrium. The oesophagus is then intubated with a flexible fibre-optic gastroscope which is passed to the stomach. The stomach is held with a laparoscopic grasper and air is carefully insufflated endoscopically. The stomach is held up to the anterior abdominal wall and a needle is passed into its lumen under endoscopic and

laparoscopic vision (Figure 6). The wire or string is passed through the needle to the stomach, grasped and withdrawn through the mouth for attachment to the PEG tube and pulled back down into position as per Gauderer-Ponsky (Charlesworth et al. 2010).
Whilst the substantial benefits of this procedure are that neighbouring viscera can be clearly seen and thus avoided and the position of the site for PEG can be carefully chosen, the major potential pitfall is insufflation of too much air into the stomach prior to having laparoscopic control of the organ. In this scenario the proximal small bowel may dilate and obscure the laparoscopic view, potentially necessitating conversion to open gastrostomy formation.
The technique for insertion of PEG at the end of a laparoscopic anti-reflux procedure is similar to that described here. The obvious concern is that pulling a PEG tube and retaining disc through a freshly made fundoplication may impact on the safety and efficacy of the initial procedure. In our series of 20 patients undergoing laparoscopic fundoplication and placement of FREKA® PEG we demonstrated no obvious adverse impact of this procedure when compared to laparoscopic fundoplication alone. The placement, or indeed re-placement, of a PEG at the conclusion of an anti-reflux procedure is occasionally mandated, particularly in neuro-developmentally delayed children, as it is safe and does not appear to impact on the efficacy of the fundoplication (Barber et al. 2009).

6.3 Primary Button

All the PEG insertion techniques described thus far involve an internal retaining disc, this usually precludes removal in the awake child and many surgeons routinely change the PEG to a balloon gastrostomy device (either Gastrostomy tube or Button) under anaesthetic some months, even up to two years, after the initial PEG placement. In order to avoid this first change of PEG to balloon device there has been a move in recent years toward primary placement of cage or balloon type button gastrostomy devices. (Figure 7)

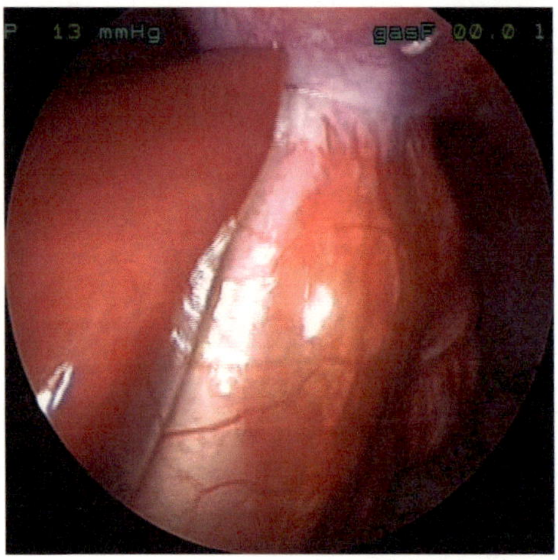

Fig. 7. Laparoscopic assisted primary Button gastrostomy placement in a newborn with oesophageal atresia without fistula

This technique was first presented in 1999. It involves placement of an umbilical laparoscopic camera port and a single (5mm) left upper quadrant working port placed under direct vision. A stitch is passed into the working port and an instrument is passed

down after it. The traction stitch is placed through the desired area of the stomach and the ends both brought out through the trocar. The trocar is then removed and if necessary the tract is dilated with a clamp, the suture is used to deliver the stomach up into the opening. Two stay sutures are placed on either side of the presenting portion and these are secured through anterior rectus fascia and are left loose until the button is in place. A single purse-string suture is placed on the stomach and a gastrostomy incision made in the centre. An appropriate button device is placed (the original description is with a balloon type gastrostomy button) and the purse-string and then the stay sutures are secured. If the wound was increased for access it is then closed. (Rothenberg et al. 1999)
The significant advantage of this procedure is the direct visualisation of the stomach and surrounding organs ensuring safety in placement. The technique as described is minimally invasive utilising only one incision in addition to the umbilical camera port, this makes it very suitable for use at the end of a laparoscopic procedure where-by an appropriately sited port-site can be used for gastrostomy placement. (Figure 8)

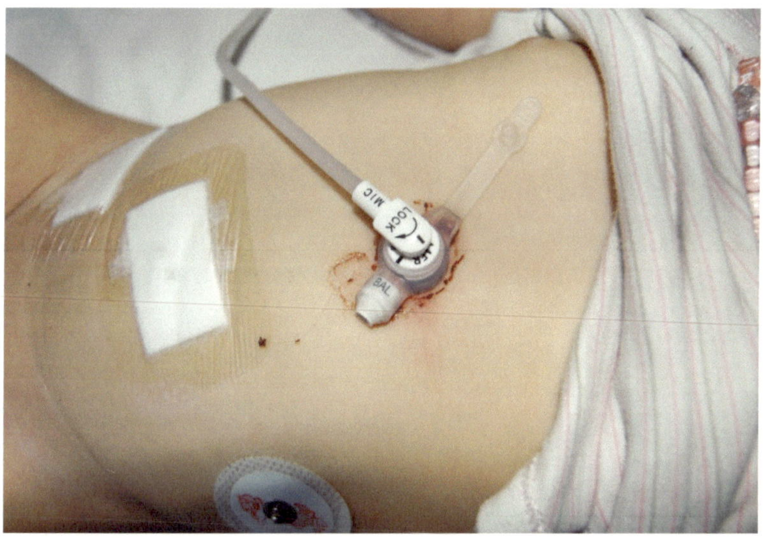

Fig. 8. Complex patient with Kabuki's Syndrome with lap assisted primary button placement. Patient underwent right nephrectomy and repair of right diaphragmatic eventration under the same anaesthetic

The associated complications in this group are certainly similar to most gastrostomy placement methods. Early displacement of the gastrostomy button, however, should be easy to manage since the stomach is well apposed to the abdominal wall with sutures. Never-the-less it is wise to ensure any early replacement tube or button is intra-luminal either endoscopically or with water-soluble contrast fluoroscopy.

6.4 Radiologically placed gastrostomy

Radiologically Placed Gastrostomy (RPG) is a developing field driven mainly by the increasing demand for gastrostomy placement in adults. It has the significant advantage of requiring no anaesthetic and no tubes or wires need to be passed down the oesophagus. This is particularly helpful in the group of patients with head, neck or oesophageal tumours.

Its utility in children remains largely unproven, due to the increased requirement for anaesthesia for interventions in children removing one of the factors that recommend RPG. The reported complication rates in adults do appear significantly lower than for surgical gastrostomy techniques and we should consider whether there is a greater role for RPG in children. (Given et al. 2004)

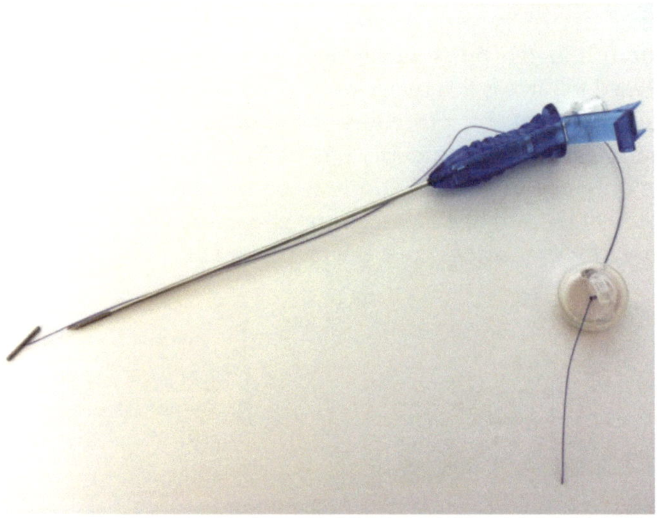

(a)

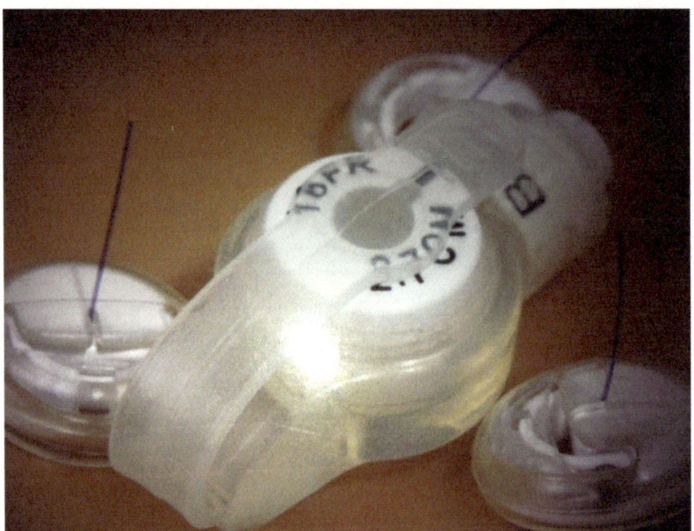

(b)

Fig. 9. The MIC-KEY® percutaneous gastropexy T-fastener and example of its use with a gastrostomy button for either radiological or endoscopic placement

Whilst the methods described for PEG placement have included a "pull technique"; RPG, in common with primary buttons and laparoscopic gastrostomy placement, requires a "push technique". This means that a wire being passed into the stomach through the anterior abdominal wall is used as a conduit for dilatation and subsequent passage of the gastrostomy device. It is possible, but more complex, to perform a "pull technique" RPG and it requires 2 operators. For safety it is widely practised that the patient being fasted for this procedure is given a quantity of dilute barium 12 hours prior so as to outline the colon. It is usual to perform a localised gastropexy with percutaneous T-fasteners (Figure 9) prior to insertion of the gastrostomy to ensure that the stomach wall remains approximated to the anterior abdominal wall.

One of the advantages of these techniques is that placement of gastro-jejunostomy tubes as a primary procedure is possible. As remarked earlier in this chapter the utility of such tubes is up for debate, however if one does wish to place such a tube the modifications to the technique above are not major and there is a relatively high success rate (Given et al. 2005).

7. Conclusion

The history of gastrostomy is very long and there has been very significant progress since the introduction of the Percutaneous Endoscopic Gastrostomy in 1979. More recent developments in minimal access surgery have driven the production of new devices and description of new techniques further and faster still. The benefits to our young patients have been significant and our ability to treat more complex and more difficult cases has been greatly aided by this process.

8. Acknowledgment

We are grateful to the parents who consented to photographs of their children appearing in this chapter.

9. References

Barber, N., Carden, C. & Mahomed, A., 2009. Does the placement of a FRECA gastrostomy at the time of laparoscopic fundoplication impact on outcome? *Surgical endoscopy*, 23(3), pp.598-601.

Borkowski, S., 1998. PEDIATRIC STOMAS, TUBES, AND APPLIANCES. *Pediatric Clinics of North America*, 45(6), pp.1419-1435.

Charlesworth, P., Hallows, M. & van der Avoirt, A., 2010. Single-Center Experience of Laparoscopically Assisted Percutaneous Endoscopic Gastrostomy Placement. *Journal of Laparoendoscopic & Advanced Surgical Techniques*, 20(1), pp.73-75.

Chung, D.H. & Georgeson, K.E., 1998. Fundoplication and gastrostomy. *Seminars in pediatric surgery*, 7(4), pp.213-9.

Cook, R., 1969. Gastrocolic fistula: A complication of gastrostomy in infancy. *Journal of Pediatric Surgery*, 4(3), p.346–349.

Cunha, F., 1946. Gastrostomy: Its inception and evolution. *The American Journal of Surgery*, 72(4), pp.610-634.

Fröhlich, T. et al., 2010. Review article: percutaneous endoscopic gastrostomy in infants and children. *Alimentary pharmacology & therapeutics*, 31(8), pp.788-801.

Gauderer, M.W., 1992. Gastrostomy techniques and devices. *The Surgical clinics of North America*, 72(6), pp.1285-98.

Gauderer, M.W., Ponsky, J.L. & Izant, R.J., 1980. Gastrostomy without laparotomy: a percutaneous endoscopic technique. 1980. *Journal of Pediatric Surgery*, 15(6), pp.872-875.

Georgeson, K.E., 1997. Laparoscopic versus open procedures for long-term enteral access. *Nutrition in clinical practice : official publication of the American Society for Parenteral and Enteral Nutrition*, 12(1 Suppl), pp.S7-8.

Given, M.F., Hanson, J.J. & Lee, M.J., 2005. Interventional radiology techniques for provision of enteral feeding. *Cardiovascular and interventional radiology*, 28(6), pp.692-703.

Given, M.F., Lyon, S.M. & Lee, M.J., 2004. The role of the interventional radiologist in enteral alimentation. *European radiology*, 14(1), pp.38-47.

Godbole, P. et al., 2002. Limitations and uses of gastrojejunal feeding tubes. *Archives of disease in childhood*, 86(2), pp.134-7.

Lo, C. et al., 2005. Consensus Statement; ESPEN guidelines on Artificial enteral nutrition - percutaneous endoscopic gastrostomy (PEG). *Clinical Nutrition*, 24(5), pp.848-861.

Rothenberg, S.S., Bealer, J.F. & Chang, J.H.T., 1999. Primary laparoscopic placement of gastrostomy buttons for feeding tubes. *Journal of Pediatric Surgery*, (March), pp.995-997.

Stringel, B.G., Geller, E.R. & L, M.S., 1995. Laparoscopic-Assisted Percutaneous Endoscopic Gastrostomy. *New York*, 8(8), pp.1209-1210.

Stringel, G., Robinson, E. & Maisel, S., 1993. Laparoscopic gastrostomy. *Pediatric Surgery International*, 8(5), pp.382-384-384.

Vervloessem, D. et al., 2009. Percutaneous endoscopic gastrostomy (PEG) in children is not a minor procedure: risk factors for major complications. *Seminars in pediatric surgery*, 18(2), pp.93-7.

2

Gastrostomy in Pediatric Patients

Brian W. Gray, Ana Ruzic and George B. Mychaliska
University of Michigan, Section of Pediatric Surgery, C.S. Mott Children's Hospital
USA

1. Introduction

Gastrostomy is one of the most common procedures performed in the pediatric population. The first gastrostomy was performed over 150 years ago, with the first successful attempts in children occurring in the late 1800's. [1] The procedure and its use in Pediatric Surgery have significantly evolved over the past several decades with the introduction of endoscopic and laparoscopic techniques to surgical practice. [2-7] These advances have resulted in the ability to perform these operations quickly, safely, and minimally invasively, while also expanding the applications for gastrostomy.

The primary indication for gastrostomy in infants and children is the need for long-term (>3-6 months) primary or supplemental enteral feeding (Table 1). This group can be subdivided into the two most common groups of gastrostomy tube candidates: those with severe dysphagia and those with failure to thrive (FTT). Most of these children with severe dysphagia have neurologic dysfunction that impairs normal swallowing. Potential sources of FTT include short gut syndrome, GI malabsorption, malignancy, trauma, chronic lung disease, and congenital heart disease, among others. Gastrostomy may also be considered in patients with pulmonary disease due to frequent aspiration of oral feeds. Rarely, a child can require gastrostomy to administer a non-palatable diet or medication. Finally, for children with primary GI abnormalities, gastrostomy placement may be a preferred means of gastric decompression.

Severe Dysphagia	***Frequent Aspiration (documented)***
Neurologic Impairment	Leading to Pulmonary Disease
Failure to Thrive	***Non-palatable Diet or Medication***
Short Gut Syndrome	Chronic renal failure diet
GI Malabsorption	HAART therapy for HIV
Malignancy	Cholestyramine for Alagille Syndrome
Trauma	
Chronic Pulmonary Disease, e.g. CF	***Gastric Decompression***
Congenital Heart Disease	Esophageal atresia with distal TEF

Table 1. Indications for Gastrostomy in Children and Infants

2. Preoperative workup

Prior to planning the operative approach to gastrostomy tube placement, one must assure the patient is indeed an appropriate candidate for such a procedure. Clinical indications, as well as anatomic and physiologic factors should be considered. Specifically, identifying a need for concomitant anti-reflux procedure dictates further pre-operative work-up. Practices vary, but in general, surgeons employ a combination of an upper gastrointestinal (UGI) study, pH probe, gastric emptying study, and in some cases endoscopy. Overuse of these resources has recently been scrutinized, largely due to poorly demonstrated utility of an UGI to evaluate GERD and therefore predict a need for an anti-reflux intervention. Consequently, a number of recent publications began advocating selective use of radiologic studies and only in cases when they were highly suspected to change the operative intervention. [8-10] In these cases, a focused history and physical exam are essential, designed to elicit symptoms of GERD and gastric feeding intolerance.

Although the sensitivity of an UGI to assess GERD is low, it remains the most utilized pre-operative modality in evaluation of patients for gastrostomy tube placement. Anatomic anomalies including malrotation, delayed gastric emptying, or esophageal stricture will alter the operative plan. Clinical evidence of severe GERD, may be difficult to obtain from some patients, and precipitates additional testing including a 24-hour pH probe. This is particularly true for the severely neurologically impaired (NI) population, which is traditionally felt to be at high risk of symptomatic GERD. Recent literature, however, challenges this notion as well, demonstrating only a 5-7% conversion rate to an antireflux operation, following initial gastrostomy in properly selected patients. [11,12,9] Finally, evidence of delayed gastric emptying may lead to placement of a gastro-jejunostomy tubes, allowing for gastric drainage via the gastric limb, while feeding via the jejunostomy limb.

In children with severe respiratory compromise, failure to thrive is common. These patients are some of the most frequent candidates for a gastrostomy tube, but also a population which presents a particular challenge in pre-operative planning. It is commonly unclear whether GERD precipitates and worsens their respiratory symptoms. In addition to the NI population, these children are most often submitted to additional pre-operative testing, including a 24-hour pH probe. Currently, the pH probe is considered the gold standard for establishing the diagnosis of GERD. [13] In most institutions, pediatric testing requires an overnight inpatient stay. A naso-esophageal probe is inserted, terminating approximately 2.5-3 cm above the lower esophageal sphincter. Continued measurements of the pH are recorded, with pH ≤ 4 indicating reflux of gastric contents. Both frequency and duration of GER are measured, as well as number of GER episodes lasting > 5 minutes, duration of the longest episode, and percentage of time esophageal pH remains ≤ 4. All of these components are then factored into a composite score (known as the DeMeester score). Values of more than 14.7 indicate pathologic GER and a need for a concomitant antireflux operation. [14]

Endoscopy is rarely used in the pediatric population solely for pre-operative evaluation prior to gastrostomy tube placement. It is a valuable tool, however, particularly when radiologic studies and history provide an inconclusive picture. Endoscopy can reliably demonstrate esophageal, gastric and duodenal ulcerations, esophagitis or gastritis, polyps, stricture or diverticula, all of which can account for feeding intolerance. Although many of these findings do not preclude placement of a gastrostomy tube, their symptoms can be identical to those of GERD. When identified, they can help establish a correct diagnosis and obviate the need for a concomitant anti-reflux procedure.

3. Gastrostomy techniques

3.1 Open/Stamm gastrostomy

The technique for a classic open, or Stamm, gastrostomy was first described by Dr. Martin Stamm in 1894. Compared with other methods for creating a gastrostomy, the Stamm technique is being used with decreasing frequency due to its invasive nature. Indications for Stamm gastrostomy include altered anatomy, history of multiple abdominal operations, an unstable patient, and concurrent laparotomy for other reasons.

Several different small open incisions can be used for a Stamm gastrostomy. These include a small vertical incision in the midline half way between the umbilicus and the xiphoid process, a left oblique subcostal incision, or a left supraumbilical transverse incision. The subcutaneous tissue and abdominal wall is divided using electrocautery. The anterior portion of the stomach is identified and a suitable anatomic location for the gastrostomy is identified. The gastrostomy should be placed in a dependent portion of the anterior wall of the stomach near the greater curvature. The gastrostomy location should be sufficiently far away from the fundus if a subsequent fundoplication is necessary. However, the position should also be sufficiently far away from the pylorus to prevent possible pyloric obstruction from an inflated gastrostomy balloon. Two concentric purse string sutures are placed using absorbable suture. Next, a small incision is made on the abdominal wall several centimeters from the original incision. Kocher clamps are placed at the edge of the fascia and a tonsil clamp is placed retrograde through the abdominal wall. A gastrostomy tube is then pulled through the tract. Balloon and mushroom tips catheters and low-profile MIC-KEY buttons (Kimberly-Clark Worldwide, Inc) have all been used in Stamm gastrostomies. Some centers place a traditional gastrostomy tube at first, while others prefer the initial placement of a MIC-KEY button. A gastrotomy is then performed in the central portion of the double purse string sutures. The gastrostomy tube is placed in the stomach, and the balloon is inflated. The purse strings are tied down to secure the gastric serosa around the tube, and the stomach is then sutured to the anterior abdominal wall with interrupted absorbable suture in four quadrants. The small abdominal wall incision is closed with a running vicryl suture. The skin is closed with a subcuticular stitch. Dressings are applied.

3.2 Laparoscopic gastrostomy

Laparoscopic gastrostomy tube placement is one of the most popular methods currently used in the pediatric population, particular for smaller children. Advantages of this technique include the use of small incisions and direct visualization of the stomach upon tube insertion to avoid hollow viscus injury. A review from our institution in 2010 found a slightly lower complication rate for laparoscopic gastrostomy compared to PEG tube placement. [15] One disadvantage is that it can be challenging to bring up the stomach through the thicker abdominal wall (>2cm thick) of larger children, so laparoscopic gastrostomy tube placement is generally reserved for younger, smaller children.

To perform a laparoscopic gastrostomy, the abdomen is prepped and draped in the usual sterile fashion. Prior to insufflation, the costal margin is marked and the proposed optimal location for the gastrostomy tube in the left upper quadrant is marked. The optimal position is at least two centimeters from the costal margin in a paramedian plane. A small incision is made in the umbilicus, the abdomen is inflated with carbon dioxide, and a five millimeter trocar is inserted. A five millimeter, thirty degree laparoscope is inserted. At this time, the patient's stomach is decompressed with an orogastric tube. A small incision is made in the left upper quadrant in the intended position for the gastrostomy tube. Care should be taken to avoid making the incision too close to the costal margin to avoid chronic pain from the tube. A five millimeter trocar is then inserted through this incision. As in the Stamm gastrostomy, the optimal location for the gastrostomy tube is a dependent portion of the stomach near the greater curvature, sufficiently far away from the pylorus. This is grasped with an atraumatic grasper through the left upper quadrant trocar and, under direct vision, brought toward the anterior abdominal wall. The abdomen is desufflated, the trocar is removed, and a portion of the stomach brought through the small incision. A silk suture is then placed through the tip of the stomach. The stomach is then secured to the fascia in four quadrants with an absorbable suture, and a single purse string is placed using absorbable suture. A gastrotomy is performed sharply or with cautery. A gastrostomy tube is then inserted directly into the stomach, and the balloon is inflated. Again, a low-profile MIC-KEY button may be placed during the initial procedure. The abdomen is re-insufflated and the laparoscope is placed through the umbilical port to confirm proper tube position. The umbilical incision is closed with an interrupted absorbable figure-of-eight suture, and the skin is closed with a subcuticular stitch. Dressings are applied.

3.3 Percutaneous Endoscopic Gastrostomy (PEG)

The PEG procedure for gastrostomy placement was developed in 1980 by Dr. Michael Gauderer as a less invasive technique of feeding tube placement for children. [16] Since that time, it has been adopted worldwide as the primary method of gastrostomy placement in adults and older children. Whereas many adults can tolerate the procedure under conscious sedation, most children still require general anesthesia for PEG placement.

PEG placement begins with placing the patient in a supine position and prepping the patient's abdomen in a usual sterile fashion. Most standard PEG kits are equipped with a sterile drape that may be used to drape the abdomen. A flexible endoscope is then inserted through the patient's mouth and guided into the stomach. For most patients, a pediatric endoscope may be used, but larger children may require an adult scope. The stomach is then insufflated, but not over-inflated. An under-inflated stomach can allow the transverse colon to become interposed between the stomach and the abdominal wall, and an over-insufflation can cause inflation of the small bowel, increasing the risk of hollow viscus injury.

The surgeon at the abdomen then chooses a proper gastrostomy site under the left costal margin at least two centimeters from the margin and depresses the skin, so that the endoscopist can identify the indentation in the anterior gastric wall. The endoscopist then illuminates the anterior gastric wall along the greater curvature, and the surgeon verifies transillumination on the abdominal wall. If clear indentation transillumination cannot be attained, then another method of gastrostomy tube placement should be pursued due to the risk of hollow viscus injury. Once a site of clear transillumination is found on the abdominal wall in a proper gastrostomy site, the surgeon then infuses local anesthetic in the skin and subcutaneous tissue. A large bore needle is then inserted through the skin into the stomach. The endoscopist then advances a polypectomy snare through the endoscope and places the snare around the end of the needle. The surgeon then inserts a looped wire through the needle. This wire is enclosed in the polypectomy snare and pulled gently out through the mouth along with the endoscope. At this point, the wire marks the tract from the mouth to the future gastrostomy site. The surgeon now makes an 8-10mm incision through the abdominal skin on either side of the wire. Next, the endoscopist attaches the steel wire loop to the tapered end of the gastrostomy tube, and the surgeon carefully pulls the abdominal end of the steel wire, gently pulling the gastrostomy tube through the mouth, esophagus, stomach, and abdominal wall. The internal gastric retainer on the gastrostomy tube should fit snugly against the anterior gastric wall. The endoscope is re-inserted into the stomach at this point to verify internal tube positioning. An external bolster and immobilizing ring are then slid over the tube to secure it into place. Care is taken to not put excessive pressure across the gastric and abdominal walls to prevent post-procedure pain and tissue necrosis. Finally, the tube is cut to the desired length, and a feeding adapter is applied to the end of the tube. No sutures are required. The PEG tube is usually changed to a low-profile button after at least six weeks to allow for tract maturation.

3.4 Laparoscopic PEG

Several studies have shown lower incidence of injury to the small and large bowel during laparoscopic gastrostomy compared to the PEG procedure. [6,15,17] The primary reason for this difference is the direct visualization of the interface between the gastric and abdominal walls that the laparoscopic technique allows. Unfortunately, the laparoscopic gastrostomy cannot be performed on children with thicker abdominal walls. For this reason, our group is increasingly performing a laparoscopic PEG procedure. Other indications include failed attempts at a traditional PEG, altered abdominal anatomy from previous surgery, and gastrostomy placement at the conclusion of a laparoscopic operation, such as Nissen fundoplication. [4,7]

The laparoscopic PEG technique is a hybrid of the laparoscopic and percutaneous techniques. The patient's abdomen is prepped in a normal and sterile fashion, and a single five millimeter laparoscopic trocar is inserted through the umbilicus. The abdomen is moderately insufflated to allow visualization of the stomach. A standard PEG procedure as described above is then completed under direct intra-abdominal visualization to prevent hollow viscus injury. As the stomach is insufflated, the abdominal cavity is desufflated after adequate visualization. An advantage of this technique is that the gastrostomy can be placed in the ideal position on the greater curvature of the stomach between the body and the antrum. If the surgeon wishes to secure the stomach to the abdominal wall, two to four t-fasteners can be placed percutaneously through the gastric wall under laparoscopic visualization. Alternatively, the surgeon has the option of suturing the gastric wall to the abdominal wall intracorporeally, but this requires placement of two additional five millimeter ports. We have not found this to be necessary in our experience. As with PEG tubes in children, laparoscopic PEGs are usually changed to a low-profile button in a separate procedure at least six weeks after initial placement.

3.5 Image-guided percutaneous gastrostomy

A recent advance in minimally invasive gastrostomy is the percutaneous placement of a gastrostomy tube under fluoroscopic guidance. This technique is performed by interventional radiologists or surgeons with advanced training in interventional radiology. The ideal patient is one without complex abdominal anatomy or previous abdominal surgery. The technique involves insufflating the stomach using an NG tube under fluoroscopic visualization. A needle is then advanced into the stomach using fluoroscopy, with entry into the lumen verified by contrast injection. A t-fastener is advanced through the needle to keep the stomach adhered to the anterior abdominal wall. A total of two to four t-fasteners are used to secure the stomach. A needle is then advanced into the stomach through the center of the t-fasteners, and its location is verified by contrast injection. Next, a wire is advanced through the needle into the stomach, and the tract is dilated using the Seldinger technique. Once the tract is sufficiently dilated, a pigtail or balloon type gastrostomy tube is advanced into the stomach, and positioning is again verified by contrast injection. Finally, the t-fasteners are tied externally over bolsters. These fasteners can be cut between three and seven days post-procedure. As with other gastrostomy tubes, feeding is usually initiated within twenty-four hours of tube placement. One large study comparing outcomes between PEG and image-guided gastrostomy found low rates of major complications in both groups, but significantly less complications in the PEG group. [18] This indicates that image-guided percutaneous gastrostomy should not be the standard of care for feeding tube placement at this time.

4. Postoperative care

Feeding through a new gastrostomy tube may begin within the first twelve to twenty-four hours after placement, barring other complicating factors, such as postoperative ileus after larger operations. Tube feeds are initiated slowly and then advanced to goal rate by the second postoperative day, or as tolerated by the patient. It is important to keep the patient's skin clean and dry by preventing leakage of gastric contents onto the skin. This can be done by keeping the external bolster snug, but not too tight, against the skin and securing the tube at a perpendicular angle to the abdominal wall. Keeping the tube perpendicular at the skin decreases the amount of soft tissue stretching encountered at the gastrostomy site. Finally, the area around the gastrostomy tube should be cleansed on a daily basis with soap and water starting forty-eight hours after surgery. These children should receive close follow-up after gastrostomy placement due to the risk of several catheter-related complications.

5. Complications

Although a common pediatric surgery procedure, gastrostomy tube placement can have serious associated complications. Early recognition, aided by a high index of suspicion, allows for prompt intervention and prevention of catastrophic sequelae. Intraoperative, early postoperative, and remote complications have all been described. [19] Knowing their timeline, as well as presentation, guides further investigations and therapy. Table 2 outlines the specific complications and the timeline in which they generally occur.

Regardless of the operative technique, hollow viscus injury, liver injury, bleeding, and malposition of the tube can occur during the creation of gastrostomy. If recognized at the time of the operation, they can be addressed immediately, preventing serious post-operative complications, including hemodynamic instability, peritonitis, and sepsis. Early post-operative complications, however, have a more subtle presentation and require a high index of suspicion. Often they are not recognized until initiation of feeds. Their symptoms vary and range from early feeding intolerance and ileus, to worsening abdominal pain, peritonitis, and signs of systemic infection. Abdominal X-rays, G-tube studies, and UGI studies can show pneumoperitoneum suggesting separation of the stomach from the abdominal wall, intraperitoneal leak from tube dislodgment, and small or large bowel injury. Contrast studies are also useful in demonstrating appropriate intra-luminal position of tube, gastric outlet obstruction from tube migration, and gastro-colonic fistulae. Some studies have shown laparoscopic placement to be associated with less complications than PEG because of direct visualization of the stomach and greater ability to secure the stomach to the anterior abdominal wall. [15]

Less severe remote complications result in frequent outpatient evaluations following the initial post-operative visit. Granulation tissue formation, tube erosion, and skin ulceration produce significant discomfort for the child, cause bleeding and leakage of the gastric contents, and lead to frequent interruption of feeds. Short of resiting the gastrostomy, the most efficient treatment of these complications is prevention. Meticulous hygiene and appropriate positioning of external tubing prevents stretching of the skin and subcutaneous tissues and subsequent enlargement of the gastrostomy tract. Parental education, both pre-operatively and post-operatively, is essential in preventing many of the skin and tract complications.

Intraoperative Complications	*Remote complications*
Hollow viscus injury	Granulation tissue formation
Liver injury	Tube erosion
Colonic placement (PEGs)	Skin ulceration
Bleeding	Intraperitoneal leak following tube exchange
Early Postoperative Complications (1-4 weeks)	Gastro-colonic fistula
Early tube dislodgment	Gastro-cutaneous fistula
Gastric separation from the abdominal wall	
Intra-peritoneal leak	
Tube occlusion	
Gastric outlet obstruction	
Surgical site infection	

Table 2. Common complications of gastrostomy tube placement

6. Conclusion

Gastrostomy tube placement in pediatric patients is a time-tested procedure that has allowed countless children the ability to attain sufficient caloric intake and thus promote healing and growth. The decision to place a gastrostomy tube is based primarily on clinical factors with ancillary testing as needed. In most patients, the tube can be removed once they demonstrate adequate oral consumption of calories to sustain continued growth and development. Once removed, the ability for the gastrostomy tract to close spontaneously appears to be dependent on the amount of time the tube was in place. One study found that tubes left in place longer than 8 months had a significantly higher chance of leaving a gastrocutaneous fistula after the gastrostomy tube was removed. [20] Some children, particularly the neurologically impaired, require an enteral feeding tube indefinitely. Advances in endoscopy and laparoscopic surgery have increased the ease of tube placement, minimized invasiveness, and decreased morbidity.

7. References

[1] Gauderer, M.W. and T.A. Stellato, *Gastrostomies: evolution, techniques, indications, and complications.* Curr Probl Surg, 1986. 23(9): p. 657-719.

[2] Jones, V.S., E.R. La Hei, and A. Shun, *Laparoscopic gastrostomy: the preferred method of gastrostomy in children.* Pediatr Surg Int, 2007. 23(11): p. 1085-9.

[3] Gauderer, M.W., *Percutaneous endoscopic gastrostomy-20 years later: a historical perspective.* J Pediatr Surg, 2001. 36(1): p. 217-9.

[4] Charlesworth, P., M. Hallows, and A. van der Avoirt, *Single-center experience of laparoscopically assisted percutaneous endoscopic gastrostomy placement.* J Laparoendosc Adv Surg Tech A. 20(1): p. 73-5.

[5] Georgeson, K.E., *Laparoscopic gastrostomy and fundoplication.* Pediatr Ann, 1993. 22(11): p. 675-7.

[6] Zamakhshary, M., et al., *Laparoscopic vs percutaneous endoscopic gastrostomy tube insertion: a new pediatric gold standard?* J Pediatr Surg, 2005. 40(5): p. 859-62.

[7] Yu, S.C., et al., *Laparoscopic-assisted percutaneous endoscopic gastrostomy in children and adolescents.* JSLS, 2005. 9(3): p. 302-4.

[8] Valusek, P.A., et al., *Does an upper gastrointestinal study change operative management for gastroesophageal reflux.* J. Pediatr Surg, 2010. 45: p. 1169-1172.

[9] Wheatley, M.J., et al., *Long-term Follow-up of Brain-Damaged Children Requiring Feeding Gastrostomy: Should an Antireflux Procedure Always Be Performed?* J Pediatr Surg, 1991. 26(3): p. 301-305

[10] Cuenca, A.G., et al., *The Usefulness of the Upper Gastrointestinal Series in the Pediatric Patient Before Anti-Reflux Procedure or Gastrostomy Tube Placement.* J Surg Res, 2011. P 1-6 (Epub ahead of print) http://www.ncbi.nlm.nih.gov/pubmed/21550057

[11] Novotny, N.M, A.L Jester, and A.P. Ladd, *Preoperative prediction of need for fundoplication before gastrostomy tube placement in children.* J Pediatr Surg, 2009. 44: p. 173-177.

[12] Kawahara, H., et al., *Should fundoplication be added at the time of gastrostomy placement in patients who are neurologically impaired?* J Pediatr Surg, 2010. 45: p. 2373-2376

[13] Soares, R.V., et al., *Interstitial Lung Disease and Gastroesophageal Reflux Disease: key role of esophageal function tests in the diagnosis and treatment.* Arq Gastroenterol, 2011. 48(2): p. 91-97.

[14] Wang, J., et al., *Composite score of reflux symptoms in diagnosis of gastroesophageal reflux disease.* World J Gastroenterol, 2004. 10(22): p. 3332-3335.

[15] Akay, B., et al., *Gastrostomy tube placement in infants and children: is there a preferred technique?* J Pediatr Surg, 2010. 45(6): p. 1147-52.

[16] Gauderer, M.W., J.L. Ponsky, and R.J. Izant, Jr., *Gastrostomy without laparotomy: a percutaneous endoscopic technique.* J Pediatr Surg, 1980. 15(6): p. 872-5.

[17] Lantz, M., H. Hultin Larsson, and E. Arnbjornsson, *Literature review comparing laparoscopic and percutaneous endoscopic gastrostomies in a pediatric population.* Int J Pediatr. 2010: p. 507616.

[18] Nah, S.A., et al., *Gastrostomy insertion in children: percutaneous endoscopic or percutaneous image-guided?* J Pediatr Surg. 45(6): p. 1153-8.

[19] Fortunato, J.E and Cuffari, C. *Outcomes of Percutaneous Endoscopy Gastrostomy in Children.* Curr Gastroenterol Rep 2011. 13: p. 293-299

[20] Gordon, J.M. and J.C. Langer, *Gastrocutaneous fistula in children after removal of gastrostomy tube: incidence and predictive factors.* J Pediatr Surg, 1999. 34(9): p. 1345-6.

3

Percutaneous Endoscopic Gastrostomy in Pediatric Patients

Omar I. Saadah
Department of Pediatrics, Faculty of Medicine, King Abdulaziz University
Saudi Arabia

1. Introduction

Adequate nutrition is important in the management of children with chronic illnesses. Patients who are unwilling or unable to eat will starve. Starvation depletes tissue stores, and ultimately leads to impaired organ function and tissue structure. Appropriate caloric intake enables growth, promotes tissue repair, and improve immune function.
Access to the intestinal tract may be via a nasal tube or by the percutaneous route, with delivery to the stomach or jejunum. Nasogastric tubes are employed for short- term feeding, usually up to four weeks. In children requiring long term tube feeding, nasogastric feeding may be uncomfortable, disfiguring and often traumatic. Percutaneous access is usually by either endoscopic or radiological techniques. Percutaneous gastrostomy is basically a sutureless approximation of the stomach to the abdominal wall. The percutaneous endoscopic gastrostomy (PEG) becomes the most popular technique nowadays.
The first PEG was performed in the pediatric operating room of University Hospitals of Cleveland on June 12, 1979 on a four-and-half-month-old child with inadequate oral intake. The procedure was performed under sedation and local anesthesia. The child did remarkably well. However, because the initial tube used was a 12F catheter with small mushroom head, external migration ensued after 3 weeks. The catheter was changed under direct visualization, using a small laparotomy (Gauderer, 2002). Since then the procedure has been adopted worldwide for both children and adults.
Because the procedure is considered minimally invasive, rapid, and associated with low risk of complications, and short hospital stay, it has become the preferred method for delivering nutritional support in vulnerable pediatric patients. The benefits not only include successful nutritional rehabilitation, but also accelerated growth (Craig et al., 2006, Sullivan et al., 2005) enhanced carer satisfaction (Avitsland et al., 2006) and quality of life (Sullivan et al., 2004).

2. Indications

The main clinical indications for PEG placement in children are as follows (Table 1):

2.1 Inability to swallow

Children with neurological impairment comprise the majority of this category. They often have difficulty eating and drinking. These difficulties are due to problems with oropharyngeal control (Gisel et al., 1998, Reilly and Skuse, 1992) and esophageal motility (Ross et al., 1988, Heikenen et al., 1999, Fonkalsrud et al., 1995), related gastro-esophageal reflux (Ross et al., 1988), and the high risk of aspiration of food and fluids into the lungs (Rogers et al., 1994, Morton et al., 1999, Taylor et al., 1994). Among the consequences for these feeding difficulties are undernutrition (Stallings et al., 1993, Sullivan et al., 2000), esophagitis (Sondheimer and Morris, 1979), recurrent chest infections (Morton et al., 1999), and progressive lung disease (Taylor et al., 1994). Much of this feeding difficulty can be overcome by giving nourishment through a gastrostomy. Unfortunately, the placement of a gastrostomy in a child with neurological impairment does carry some risk, and parents are frequently reluctant to have a gastrostomy placed (Sullivan, 1992). Families with affected children need better information when making the difficult decision about whether to accept or request a gastrostomy for their child. Most children undergoing PEG tube feeding showed improved weight gain after PEG tube feeding (Rempel et al., 1988, Shapiro et al., 1986, Sanders et al., 1990, Brant et al., 1999). Changes in rate of length growth appeared to be less predictable and occurred only in a minority of children. The improvement of physical growth coupled with improvement in the general health and the family quality of life (Stevenson, 2005). Direct aspiration of orally ingested material and saliva may be a reason for recommending PEG tube feeding (Brant et al., 1999, Sulaeman et al., 1998). But gastro-esophageal reflux is also thought to contribute to aspiration indirectly (Morton et al., 1999). Both gastro-esophageal reflux and aspiration can occur without symptoms (Rogers et al., 1994) and the investigations that are often used to diagnose gastro-esophageal reflux appear to be unreliable. Therefore, the decision of anti-reflux procedure together with gastrostomy may not be easy unless a child's symptoms are severe despite appropriate medications (Puntis et al., 2000, Sullivan, 1999).

Clinical indications	
1.	Inability to swallow, most commonly neurologically impaired children
2.	Chronic illnesses with inadequate caloric intake
	Chronic renal failure
	Cystic fibrosis
	Congenital heart disease
	Childhood cancer
	Human immune deficiency virus infection (HIV)
	Crohn's disease
3.	Unpalatable medication
4.	Permanent enteral access and gastric decompression

Table 1. Indications for PEG insertion

2.2 Chronic illnesses with inadequate intake

Children with chronic illnesses are usually anorexic, have increased metabolic demands and usually cachectic. Children with the following conditions fall under this category:

2.2.1 Chronic renal disease

Chronic renal disease is characterized by a predisposition to anorexia and vomiting. Poor appetite may be due to abnormal taste sensation (Bellisle et al., 1995), the requirement for multiple medications, the preference for water in the polyuric child, and elevated level of circulating cytokines, which act through the hypothalamus to affect appetite and satiety (Mak et al., 2006). Vomiting may result from gastro-esophageal reflux and delayed gastric emptying in association with increased polypeptide hormones (Ravelli et al., 1992).

When the caloric and protein intake become insufficient to maintain growth despite dietary manipulation and medication (Rees and Shaw, 2007), enteral feeding is preferred through a gastrostomy. Enteral feeding can allow catch-up growth even in infants and young children with severe chronic renal failure (Kari et al., 2000). It is better to place the PEG tube prior to commencement of peritoneal dialysis in order to decrease the risk of fungal peritonitis (von Schnakenburg et al., 2006).

Children on dialysis have even more problems that affect their nutritional intake. Such children are likely to be on fluid restriction, the presence of full abdomen due to indwelling dialysate in patients on peritoneal dialysis may affect their appetite, and there may be considerable loss of protein in the dialysate.

Children with chronic renal failure, post renal transplantation tends to improve their appetite, and they succeed in the transition to oral feeding, therefore it becomes possible to remove the PEG tube (Ledermann, 2005, Pugh and Watson, 2006).

2.2.2 Cystic fibrosis

Children with cystic fibrosis (CF) commonly fail to thrive due to increased resting energy expenditure (Buchdahl et al., 1988), associated anorexia (Shepherd et al., 1980), increased energy requirements associated with chronic respiratory infection (Lapey et al., 1974, Kraemer et al., 1978), maldigestion and malabsorption (Lapey et al., 1974).

Nutritional repletion and intervention involving prescription of energy rich food and fluids, optimization of pancreatic enzyme replacement therapy, oral supplements may be required (Anthony et al., 1999). However, in a proportion of patients, particularly those with more advanced pulmonary disease, these measures alone are insufficient to maintain body weight (Durie and Pencharz, 1992).

Few studies have assessed the efficacy of gastrostomy feeding in malnourished children with CF (Efrati et al., 2006, Truby et al., 2009, Oliver et al., 2004, Van Biervliet et al., 2004). It has been suggested that the early restoration of nutritional status may result in improved weight gain, improved response to treatment for respiratory exacerbations, amelioration of the progressive decline in lung function, extended survival, and perhaps improved quality of life.

2.2.3 Congenital heart disease

Children with heart disease often have a normal birth weight but show poor weight gain and cannot maintain their growth after birth. The cause of this thought to be multifactorial and may include factors such as inadequate caloric intake, increased oxygen consumption, hypermetabolism, reduced absorption, and feeding intolerance (Mitchell et al., 1995, Leitch, 2000). These factors reflect the need for increased energy intake, and thus the dietary intervention is often necessary to improve the nutritional status of these children.

Delivering enteral nutritional support through PEG for 15 child with congenital cardiac problems was reported to be safe with rare minor complications and no major complications, and effective in terms of improving weight gain at 4 weeks and at 6 months after PEG tube insertion (Hofner et al., 2000). The rate of gastrostomy complications was more when percutaneous radiological technique was used in 58 children with cardiac disease. Major complications included intestinal perforation (3.4%) and aspiration pneumonia (12.1%). Significant weight gain was observed despite complications (Sy et al., 2008).

2.2.4 Childhood cancer

Almost half of children with cancer experience malnutrition due to numerous tumor- and treatment-related factors (Smith et al., 1991, Sala et al., 2004). It is recognized that a diminished nutritional status may be a contributing factor for decreased immune function, delayed wound healing, and disturbed drug metabolism influencing prognosis (Bosaeus et al., 2001, Tisdale, 1997). Children with cancer are particularly vulnerable to malnutrition, because they exhibit elevated nutritional needs due to the disease and its treatment. At the same time, children have increased requirements of nutrients to attain appropriate growth and neurodevelopment (Han-Markey, 2000). It has been demonstrated that adequate nutrition is an important determinant for several clinical outcome measures such as treatment response, quality of life, and cost of care (van Eys, 1979, Rickard et al., 1986). Various types of high energy protein formulas and liquid supplements are offered to increase energy density in pediatric patients, but with less success and poor tolerance because of taste and smell perception. Children with painful severe mucositis may have problem tolerating oral feeding. A PEG is successfully used method with high acceptance by oncologists, children, and parents demonstrating improvements in weight gain and reduced family frustration due to eating problems (Skolin et al., 2002, Pedersen et al., 1999). The placement of a PEG is indicated when oral ingestion is not sufficient to cover the daily energy needs. It is rarely associated with more than minor complications. The most common complication was superficial wound infection occurred during neutropenic episodes (Skolin et al., 2002, Pedersen et al., 1999).

2.2.5 Human immunodeficiency virus (HIV) infection

Malnutrition, one of the most common and obvious signs of pediatric human immunodeficiency virus (HIV) disease, may influence the infected child's already compromised immune response. In HIV-infected children, reduced growth and lean body mass appears early (Miller et al., 1993, Halsey et al., 1990). Gastrostomy tube feedings have become a major means of nutrition in children with HIV infection when other oral methods fail (Henderson et al., 1994). HIV-infected children with higher CD4 counts and lower weight-for-height z scores are likely to respond favorably to gastrostomy tube feedings and had a 2.8-fold reduction in the risk of dying for every positive unit change in weight z score (Miller et al., 1995). The HIV-infected children who received gastrostomy tube feeding had more complications associated with the tube than has been reported in the non-HIV pediatric literature (Marin et al., 1994). The newer combination antiretroviral therapies used to treat HIV-infected children have result in dramatic delays in HIV progression, with reduction in the mortality and morbidity. However adherence to highly effective antiretroviral therapy in children may be problematic (Matsui, 1997). Reasons for non compliance include refusal, drug tolerability, and adverse reactions. PEG was suggested as a mean to administer medications to overcome such problems and improve adherence (Temple et al., 2001, Shingadia et al., 2000). PEG also significantly reduced parent reported times for medication administration and, therefore, may have the potential to improve the quality of life of HIV-infected children and their families (Shingadia et al., 2000).

2.2.6 Crohn's disease

Malnutrition and growth failure are common at presentation in children with Crohn's disease (Kirschner et al., 1978) . Nutritional rehabilitation is often an important part of the management of children with Crohn's disease, but hampered by anorexia and the unpalatability of elemental formulas commonly used in children with Crohn's disease. An elemental formula has been shown to be as effective as steroids in reducing the remission of active disease while avoiding the negative effects on growth (Sanderson et al., 1987). It has been suggested that the more palatable polymeric formulas can be used for treatment of active Crohn's disease rather than the unpalatable elemental formulas. Large amounts are required to be consumed daily with no solid food ingestion in order to achieve such therapeutic effect, and this may remain difficult to take by mouth. Nasogastric tube has been used for this reason (Belli et al., 1988), but has the advantage of being uncomfortable, disfiguring, and embarrassing for the child or adolescent if the tube left in place during the day time. A PEG can overcome this problem as it is hidden under clothing and is not visible. The use of PEG in children with Crohn's disease to deliver enteral nutrition has been reported to be safe and effective (Israel and Hassall, 1995, Pashankar and Israel, 1997, Cosgrove and Jenkins, 1997). Most of the complications of gastrostomy were minor and easily treatable. Closure of the gastrostomy tract after removal was almost complete. Only one study reported no closure of the gastrocutaneous fistula after PEG removal in one patient requiring surgical closure (Israel and Hassall, 1995). PEG remains a good and safe option if nasogastric tube feeding is not possible.

2.3 Unpalatable medications

Occasionally, PEG can be used in children with long-standing renal or cardiac failure who are dependent on large quantities of drugs for survival but resist medication provided orally (Gauderer, 2002).

2.4 Permanent enteral feeding

Patients with limited intestinal function, such as short bowel syndrome (Buchman, 2007)and intestinal pseudo-obstruction (Michaud et al., 2001) may benefit from PEG. PEG tube can also be used for gastric decompression in patients with intestinal pseudo-obstruction.

3. Contraindications

The contraindications for PEG insertion are related to conditions that cause pharyngeal or esophageal obstruction, interfere with gastrostomy site identification, or have been identified as being more likely to produce complications (Table 2).

Contraindications
Patients who are unfit for endoscopy
Pharyngeal / esophageal obstruction
Active coagulopathy
Portal hypertension with gastric varices
Severe ascites
Peritoneal dialysis
Epidermolysis bullosa
Significant kypho-scolisosis when access to the stomach may be compromised
Failure of translumination through abdominal wall or clear point of indentation

Table 2. Contraindications for PEG insertion

4. PEG placement

4.1 Technique

The 'pull' technique described by Gauderer and Stellato is recommended and is probably the technique most widely employed (**Fig.1**). After preparation of the abdomen, administration of prophylactic antibiotic and preparing the appropriate PEG equipment, under general anaesthesia, a flexible gastroscope appropriate to the size and weight of the child is passed into the stomach, which is gently insufflated. The abdominal wall is transilluminated by the endoscope. The assistant's finger then indents the anterior abdominal wall, and this indentation must be seen clearly through the endoscope to confirm close apposition of the stomach to the venteral abdominal wall. A small skin incision is made at the intended gastrostomy site. The percutaneous needle and trocar is passed directly into the stomach under endoscopic vision. The guidewire is introduced through the needle and grasped by the endoscopist's snare. The scope is gently withdrawn, bringing the guidewire with it. An appropriately sized PEG tube is looped to the thread and lubricated along its whole length to enable smooth passage through the throat and oesophagus. The thread is gently pulled back from the abdominal insertion site and the PEG placed in position. The outer flange of the tube is positioned loosely against the anterior abdominal wall. The opposition of the inner flange with the gastric wall can be checked by repeat endoscopy.

4.2 Post-operative care

Postoperatively, the child will be closely monitored. The PEG tube should not be used for 24 hours. Feeding usually start with small amount of oral rehydration solution and then gradually increased to the desired volume. It is generally best to use diluted formulas (quarter-strength or half-strength) and then advance the diet first in volume and then in concentration over 3-4 days. Inability to tolerate increased volume is evident by abdominal distension, vomiting, or increased gastric residuals. Inability to tolerate increased osmolarity is evidenced by diarrhea. Once the child is able to tolerate formula sufficiently in volume and concentration, intravenous fluids can be discontinued. Initially, bolus feeding can be delivered slowly using enteral feeding pump several times a day. Gastric residuals should be checked before application of every bolus of enteral feeding. Careful assessment of the gastric residuals may help in improving feeding tolerance and minimising the risk of pulmonaray aspiration. Children who are taking medications for seizures will have their medications converted to an intravenous form until they are able to tolerate gastric route of administration.

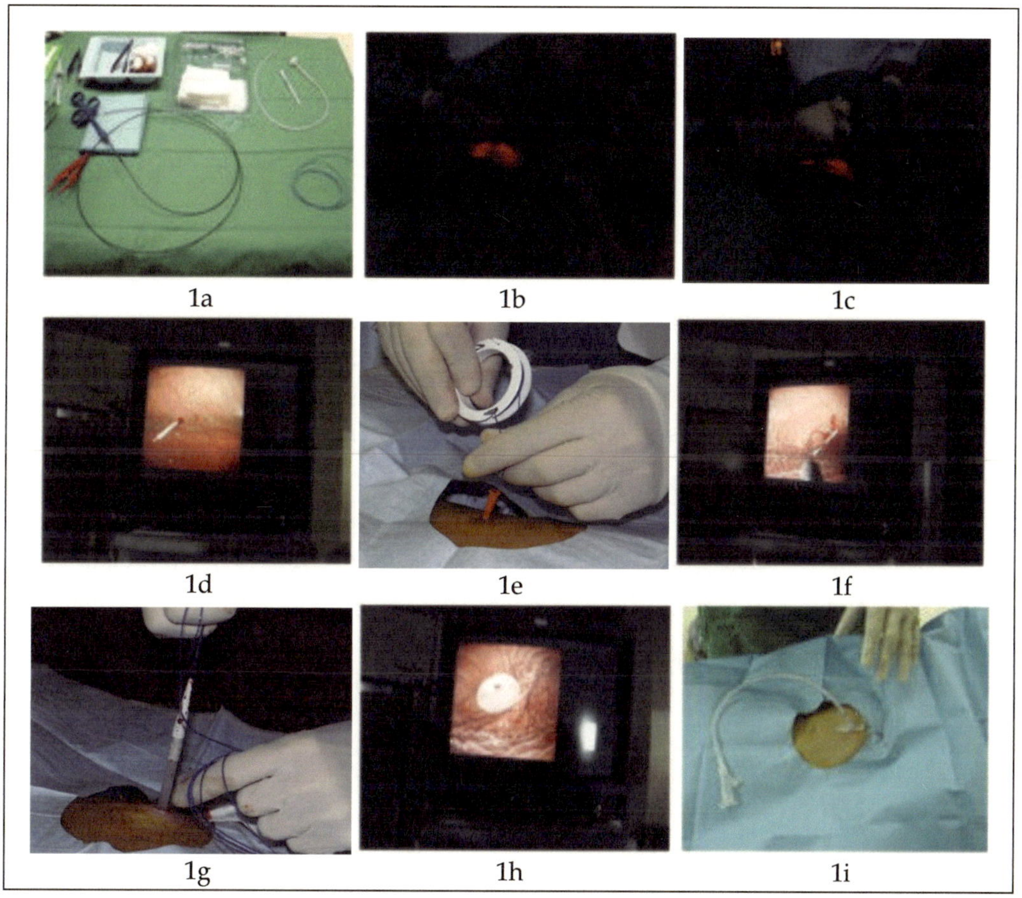

Fig. 1. The technique of PEG insertion.1a. The main PEG equipment including, a PEG tube, a guidewire, a needle with a trocar and a snare. 1b. Abdominal wall transillumination by the endoscope with testing for indentation. 1c. Making a small skin incision at the intended gastrostomy site. 1d. Passing the needle and trocar directly to the stomach under endoscopic vision. 1e. Passing the guidewire through the needle. 1f. Grasping the guidewire by the snare to bring through the mouth. 1g. Pulling the guidewire and the anchored tube back from the abdominal insertion site. 1h. Checking the opposition of the inner flange with the gastric wall. 1i. PEG tube after insertion

5. Feeding through PEG tube

In Infants less than 12 months of age, an infant formula should be used. In patients with high caloric needs or with poor tolerance to increased formula volume, the formula may be concentrated and/or modular nutrients, such as glucose polymer or lipid, may be added. Infants with Cow's milk protein allergy, gastrointestinal maldigestion or absorption, and short bowel syndrome may benefit from amino acid-based or casein-based formulas.

Older children may be offered any of the following options depending on the underlying disease and the socio-economic status:

5.1 Polymeric feeds

Polymeric feeds are the most commonly used enteral feeds. Most children will tolerate a polymeric formula. They contain whole protein as a nitrogen source and energy of 1 kcal/ml. They are lactose and gluten free. Moreover they contain enough vitamins, trace elements and essential fatty acids to prevent deficiencies. Adult formulas should be avoided because the caloric-to-nutrient ratio is inadequate for children. Their use may result in calcium, phosphorus and vitamin deficiency, especially in patients with low-caloric needs.

5.2 Elemental feeds

Elemental feeds contain either amino acid or hydrolyzed protein. They are relatively expensive with unpalatable taste. It should be used only in situations where there is profound impairment in the gastrointestinal digestive and absorptive functions.

5.3 Blenderised food

This is used in many developing countries primarily because it is cheaper than commercially prepared feeds. It is viscous and chunks of food may block the feeding tube and increase the risk of complications. Feeding contamination is a further risk that may predispose to fungal growth in the lumen of the tube **(Fig. 2)**.

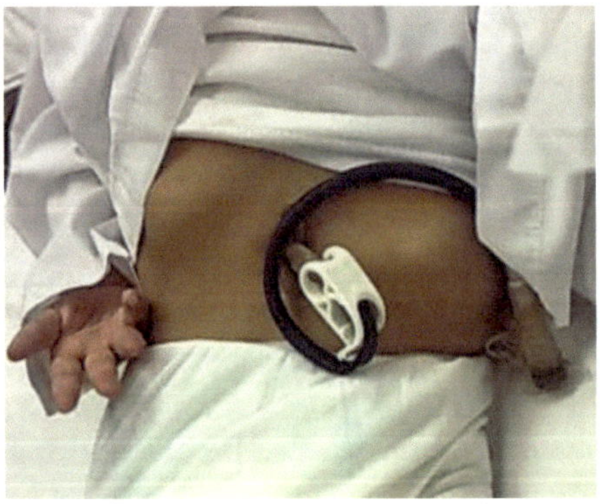

Fig. 2. Fungal contamination of the PEG tube

6. Care of the PEG tube

The care of the child with the PEG differs from that of adults, because of the child's smaller yet growing body and because nutritional needs change in time. Moreover, children, especially if chronically underfed, have very sensitive skin that must be protected effectively (Hagelgans and Janusz, 1994). Two main problems are the accurate selection of a properly sized device and then frequent checks and replacement with a more suitable size if necessary. The device should grow with the child. It must be as small as possible; both to minimize annoyance to the child, but it also must prevent leakage of gastric content or pressure necrosis and allow feeding to pass through easily.

It is important to secure the external flange of the tube nearly 3 mm above skin level (Ricciardi and Brown, 1994) to prevent leakage of the gastric content and to allow freedom of movement, which is very important for children to avoid traumatizing the gastric mucosa or pulling the bumper into the tract. It also allows air circulation to the skin around and underneath the disc to avoid pressure necrosis.

Skin care includes careful daily control of the position of the external flange with rotation and careful cleaning of the skin near the gastrostomy. It is important to protect the skin with zinc oxide cream or with absorbent powder or paste if there is any leakage (Hagelgans and Janusz, 1994).

Tube obstruction can easily occur. It is necessary to flush with 10 to 15 ml warm water before and after any introduction. You may need to flush only after feeding in very small babies. Food must be fluids such as liquid enteral formula. Medicine must be well dissolved before administration through the tube. If the tube is blocked, it should be flushed with a solution of water and half a capsule of crushed and dissolved pancreatic enzymes.

Bolus feeding must take at least 20 minutes and can be administered by a gravity flow system, by pump, or by syringe. If the child has fever or when the weather is warm, it is necessary to administer additional water, especially if the child is exclusively fed by tube.

In children with PEG oral function should always be stimulated. Babies can be provided with a dummy especially during meals while older children can be offered something to chew or suck, such as chewing gum, piece of bread etc. It can comfort them and help the anatomical and functional development of the mouth (Tawfik et al., 1997). Mouth cleaning should be performed daily to allow a healthy growth of teeth.

7. Replacement of the PEG tube

Once placed, PEG tubes are left *in situ* until signs of cracking appear, usually after 12 months. Damaged tubes need replacing; this can easily be done at bedside, with balloon gastrostomy. Initial PEG needs to be removed before replacement. PEG removal techniques are varied. PEGs may be removed endoscopically by grasping the inner flange with a snare or basket and delivering it via the oral cavity in a retrograde fashion after cutting the external tube at skin level. Alternatively, the device can be removed percutaneously by traction provided that the inner flange is collapsible. This approach precludes the need for endoscopy unless complications are anticipated or encountered. The third approach involves cutting the device at skin level and allowing the inner flange to pass via the alimentary tract (''cut and push'' technique). This is commonly performed in adult practice, but is generally thought to be unacceptable in children due to risks of esophageal and intestinal obstruction. Esophageal obstruction, perforation, mediastinitis, retropharyngeal abscess formation, gastric outlet, intestinal and ileostomy obstruction, enterocutaneous fistula formation, tract disruption and death have been variously described with PEG removal (Yaseen et al., 1996, Siegel and Douglass, 2004, Palmer et al., 2006, Mollitt et al., 1998, Lattuneddu et al., 2003, Kobak et al., 2000, El-Rifai et al., 2004). Traction removal is performed under general anesthesia in children and involves application of a significant pulling force to deliver the device in full. Dilatation of the tract may be required in some cases.

For PEG replacement, parents may prefer a skin-level gastrostomy. This option should not be considered until the PEG tube has been *in situ* for at least 3 months, ensuring that the seal between the stomach and abdominal wall is intact and thus avoiding peritoneal soiling. Different types of skin-level replacement gastrostomy tubes including Bard® mushroom-shaped tube and the MICKEY® balloon type tube (**Fig.3**) are available. These tubes differ in the manner in which they are inserted and secured to the abdominal wall. The MICKEY® tube is inserted without using a stylet, while Bard® tube is inserted with assistance of a stylet. In addition, the MICKEY® tube is secured by a balloon, while the Bard® tube is secured by a mushroom-shaped tip. The MICKEY® tube can easily be inserted at bedside without the need for endoscopy or dye study to confirm location. The Bard® tube insertion using a stylet requires some force. This may increase the risk of disrupting the fistula tract (Fox et al., 1997). It requires endoscopy or dye study for confirmation. Replacement of skin-level devices may be required if the initial device gets blocked, dislodged, or poorly secured, especially after balloon rupture when using The MICKEY® tube. When gastrostomy tube dislodged, timely replacement is important because the fistulous tract will begin to close within hours, making subsequent replacement more difficult. If commercial replacement skin-level devices are not available, a similar size Foley catheter can be temporarily inserted.

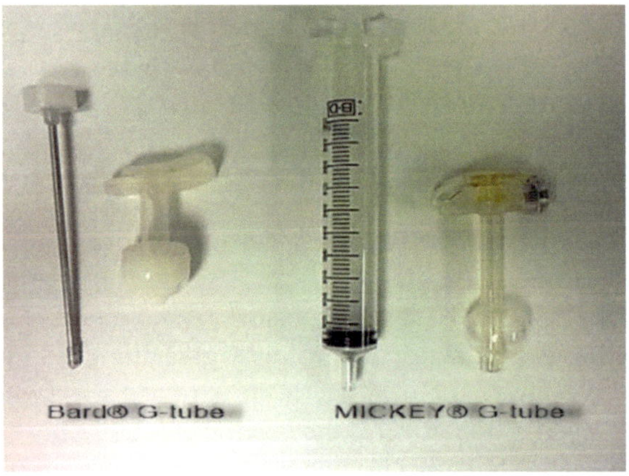

Fig. 3. Skin-level gastrostomy tubes

8. Complications of the PEG tube

The peri-operative and post-operative complications of the PEG tube are summarized in Table 3.

Complications
1. Peri-operative complications
Tension pneumoperitoneum
Peritonitis
Esophageal perforation
Intra-abdominal bleeding
2. Post-operative complications
Wound infection
Necrotizing fasciitis
Granulation tissue
Buried bumper syndrome
Tube migration
Inadvertent tube removal
Bloody PEG aspirate / hematemesis
Bowel perforation
Gastroesophageal reflux and pulmonary aspiration

Table 3. Complications of PEG insertion

8.1 Peri-operative complications

8.1.1 Tension pneumoperitoneum

Benign pneumoperitoneum is common after PEG tube insertion, with reported incidence of over 50% (Hillman, 1982, Gottfried et al., 1986, Wojtowycz et al., 1988). Conservative management of patients with pneumoperitoneum, who have undergone a recent PEG in the absence of additional symptoms, is suggested. It should be of concern if the intraabdominal air is worsening or when it is found in the presence of signs of peritonitis, portal and/or mesenteric venous gas, systemic inflammatory response and/or sepsis (Wojtowycz et al., 1988). It may occasionally be a sign of possible bowel injury (Milanchi and Allins, 2007). A tension pneumoperitoneum may occur with excessive endoscopic insufflations and a large leak occurs around the gastric needle entry site (Kealey et al., 1996).This can result in rapid respiratory embarrassment and cardiopulmonary arrest. Urgent management involves cessation of insufflations, gastric aspiration through the endoscope and peritoneal decompression via a large cannula placed percutaneously into the peritoneal cavity.

8.1.2 Peritonitis

Peritonitis occurring shortly after PEG insertion is either due to associated visceral trauma (usually colon), or due to gastric leakage because of separation of the stomach from the anterior abdominal wall (Kimber et al., 1998). Delay in making the diagnosis and institution of appropriate treatment may result in death (Lowe et al., 1997). Children with peritonitis may develop abdominal distension, guarding and generalized abdominal tenderness, with tachycardia, and pallor, and may be fever. Their clinical condition progressively deteriorates. Laparoscopy or laparotomy is warranted after stabilization for children with suspected peritonitis. PEG placement in children with chronic renal failure following initiation of peritoneal dialysis is associated with a high risk of fungal peritonitis (von Schnakenburg et al., 2006, Ledermann et al., 2002). The mortality and morbidity reported create more apprehension of recommending the PEG approach after chronic peritoneal dialysis has been initiated. At present, the evidence would favor placement of the gastrostomy early, before or preferably at the same time as peritoneal catheter insertion (Watson, 2006).

8.1.3 Esophageal perforation

Esophageal perforation is a rare complication that occurs as a result of using inappropriately large gastroscope in small infants or due to poor technique in retrieval of the guidewire especially if metallic guidewire is used (Beasley et al., 1995, Haynes et al., 1996). The presence of unrecognized esophageal stricture or abnormal fragile mucosa such as epidermolysis bullosa can be a predisposing factor for esophageal perforation (Haynes et al., 1996). This complication can be avoided with careful examination of the patient, and with using an appropriate gastroscope suitable for the age and body weight of the child. Metallic guidewires are not commonly used nowadays and being replaced with softer guidewires.

8.1.4 Intra-abdominal bleeding

PEG can be associated with life-threatening bleeding, especially when multiple needle punctures have been made. Acute hemorrhage following PEG is rarely reported (Lau and Lai, 2001, Wiggins et al., 2007). Unsussceeful passage of the needle could have caused the gastric artery branch laceration or breaches in the splenic and superior mesenteric veins or due to a liver laceration. It presents with unexplained post-procedure hypotension. Early recognition and treatment are essential.

8.2 Post-operative complications

8.2.1 Wound infection

PEG is a foreign body, and therefore creates and maintains a potential nidus for bacterial colonization. Children who require gastrostomy are often malnourished and have other medical problems that make them more susceptible to gastrostomy wound infection(**Fig. 4**). Approximately 10% of children develop erythema and tenderness at the insertion site (Khattak et al., 1998). The most common causative organism was *staphylococcus aureus* (Saadeddin et al., 2005, Ahmad et al., 2003). Children tend to harbor polymicrobial aerobic-anaerobic flora and Candida at the gastrostomy site wound infection (Brook, 1995). Factors that contribute to the development of infection may include gastric acid leakage and pressure areas from an excessively tight tube (Iber et al., 1996, Bell et al., 1995). Preventing measures including checking the position of the exteranal flange, cleaning the skin and rotating the tube daily can be followed. Meta-analysis of randomized-controlled trials of antibiotic prophylaxis prior to PEG insertion in adults (Jafri et al., 2007) has shown that prophylactic antibiotics are effective in reducing the incidence of PEG site wound infection. Both cephalosporin-based prophylaxis, such as cefazolin and penicillin-based prophylaxis, such as co-amoxiclav are equally effective. If infection diagnosed early, oral broad-spectrum antibiotics for 5-7 days may be all that is required for a PEG site infection. If there are more systemic signs, intravenous broad-spectrum antibiotics coupled with local wound care are necessary.

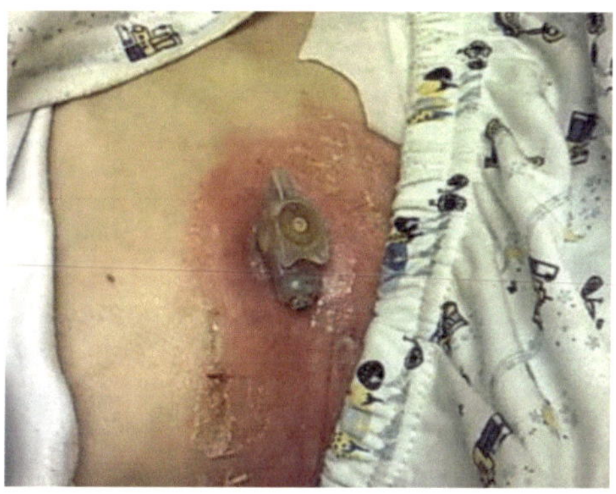

Fig. 4. Wound infection with associated cellulitis

8.2.2 Necrotizing fasciitis

A rare but potentially life-threatening complication is the development of necrotizing fasciitis. Children with pre-existing wound infections, malnutrition, and impaired immunity are at increased risk (Fox et al., 1997, Farrell et al., 1988). The microbiology of necrotizing fasciitis is complex. Multiple aerobic and anaerobic microorganisms display synergy and are responsible for the lethality of this condition (Giuliano et al., 1977). Management consists of broad spectrum intravenous antibiotics and aggressive surgical debridement.

8.2.3 Granulation tissue formation

Granulation tissue following insertion is common (**Fig.5**). It may occur in response to chronic leakage or infection. The granulation tissue can cause discharge, irritation, and discomfort. It can bleed in response to trauma. Frequent topical application of silver nitrate is often required and recurrence is common. It is important to protect the surrounding normal skin with petroleum jelly during cauterization with silver nitrate to avoid chemical burns. Daily cleaning of the stoma and rotation of the PEG tube may help in its prevention.

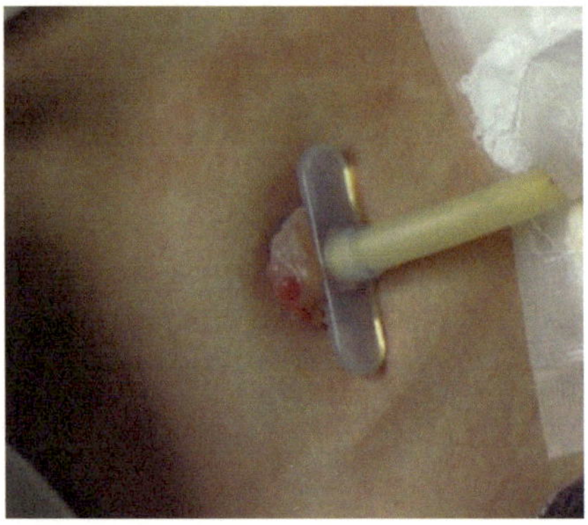

Fig. 5. Granulation tissue formation

8.2.4 Buried bumper syndrome

Buried bumper syndrome is a rare but serious complication of PEG. Published experience in children with buried bumper syndrome is very scares (Furlano et al., 2008, Kohler et al., 2008, Hodges et al., 2001). The bumper becomes lodged anywhere between the gastric wall and the skin along the PEG tract. Partial or complete growth of gastric mucosa over the internal bolster may occur. The inability to infuse the feeding formula through the tube and leakage around the tube with abdominal pain are the most common manifestation (Schwartz et al., 1989). Other symptoms that may be experienced are erythema and edema at the gastrostomy site. The endoscopic examination may reveal small irregular slit or a raised mount of the mucosa at the previous tube site. A buried bumper should be removed even if the patient is asymptomatic, because of the risk of tube impaction in the abdominal wall and/or gastric perforation. Computed tomography and ultrasonography can be helpful in localizing the bumper and in deciding the appropriate approach for removing the PEG either surgical or endoscopic. A number of approaches have been used for the treatment of buried bumper syndrome. Initial reports used incision of the skin and dissection to remove the impacted bumper, followed by insertion of the replacement tube (Shallman et al., 1988, Nelson, 1989, Lee, 1990). Another strategy involves placing a guidewire through the impacted tube, followed by pushing the impacted bumper into the stomach using dilators externally. The bumper is removed endoscopically and replacement tube is inserted through the fistula (Klein et al., 1990, Ma et al., 1995). The selected method has to be safe and should be tailored to the individual patient's needs.

8.2.5 Gastrostomy tube migration

The inner flange may enter the pylorus causing complete or partial obstruction (Hussain and Thambidorai, 2000, Berry and Vellacott, 1992). If the PEG is within mobile bowel it may act as an axis for volvulus causing intestinal obstruction (Waxman et al., 1991, Senac and

Lee, 1983). This complication occurs if the PEG has been inserted in the distal antrum, close to the pylorus. This complication can be avoided by careful placement of the PEG on the greater curve, proximal to the antrum and pyloric canal.

8.2.6 Inadvertent tube removal

PEG tract maturation usually occurs within the first 7-10 days but may be delayed up to 4 weeks in the presence of malnutrition. Inadvertent PEG tube removal can rarely occur (Larson et al., 1987, Dwyer et al., 2002). Irritable and hyperactive children are more liable to this complication. A PEG tube accidentally removed before the PEG tract maturation completed, should be replaced endoscopically. The stomach and the abdominal wall can separate from each other, resulting in free perforation. If the PEG tube is dislodged less than one month after placement, repeat endoscopy should be performed to replace the tube. When recognized early, the replacement PEG tube can be placed either near or even through the same PEG tube site (Galat et al., 1990). Blindly reinserting a new tube may lead to its placement inside the peritoneal cavity. If recognition is delayed, the patient should be kept NPO (nothing per oral), a nasogastric tube should be placed, and broad-spectrum antibiotics should be started. A new PEG should be placed after 7-10 day. Surgical exploration is indicated if signs of peritonitis/sepsis are present. A replacement tube can be placed without endoscopy through presumably mature tract, when a PEG tube dislodged more than one month after placement.

8.2.7 Bloody PEG aspirate / hematemesis

Gastrointestinal bleeding after PEG placement has been reported rarely in children (Kazi et al., 1997, Weiss et al., 1999). If the PEG flange is loose and mobile within the stomach it can irritate the gastric mucosa, and if too tight it can erode the gastric wall by pressure necrosis. Either process may lead to gastric bleeding. Most patients present with bleeding between two weeks and 6 months. Delayed presentation after 12 years from PEG placement was reported in one child. (Weiss et al., 1999). Because upper gastrointestinal bleeding is not always related to the PEG, endoscopy is recommended for diagnosis. Esophagitis and gastritis may both occur in chronically ill children, especially in neurologically impaired children with reflux esophagitis.

8.2.8 Bowel perforation

Gastro-colo-cutaneous fistulae may occur rarely when the colon is inadvertently punctured and traversed during PEG placement (Gauderer, 1991, Hacker and Cattau, 1987). Patients may present acutely with colonic perforation and peritonitis (Kimber et al., 1998). More commonly, patients present chronically with stool leaking around the PEG tube or through the stoma during tube removal or replacement. The diagnosis is made using contrast radiography via the PEG tube. In most cases, there is no evidence of intraperitoneal leakage or gastro-colic fistula. Management consists of removing the tube and allowing the fistula to close (Berger and Zarling, 1991). Should the patient develop signs of peritonitis or the fistula fail to close, surgery is often required.

To avoid this complication, the introducing needle should not be inserted into the stomach without adequate gastric insufflations, appropriate transillumination, and endoscopically visible focal indentation upon external palpation.

8.2.9 Gastroesophageal reflux and pulmonary aspiration

Gastroesophageal reflux is a common problem in neurologically impaired children (Bozkurt et al., 2004, Gangil et al., 2001). Children with symptoms of reflux who do not respond to medical therapy or with evidence of pulmonary aspiration caused by their reflux should undergo a surgical gastrostomy along with an anti-reflux procedure. In children without symptoms of reflux or with mild reflux responding well to medical treatment, an endoscopic percutaneous approach may be used. There is no role for a prophylactic anti-reflux procedure (Sulaeman et al., 1998, Khattak et al., 1998, Isch et al., 1997). The choice between a gastrostomy with or without an anti-reflux procedure has to be carefully evaluated because the failure rate and the incidence of major complications are high in neurologically impaired children undergoing anti-reflux procedure (Borgstein et al., 1994). In difficult cases, it may be useful to attempt a trial of nasogastric feeds for one month to assess tolerance before making a decision. It has been suggested that symptomatic Gastroesophageal reflux occurs frequently after PEG (Cameron et al., 1995). Pulmonary aspiration has been rarely reported in children following percutaneous gastrostomy feeding (Morton et al., 1999, Sy et al., 2008). It is unclear whether this is a consequence of the change in volume, consistency and composition of the feeds or a consequence of the procedure. If this problem occurs, medical treatment with prokinetics and changes in the formula or in the rate and volume of feeds should be attempted before restoring to an anti-reflux procedure.

9. Conclusion

PEG insertion in children who cannot achieve adequate oral intake is an established route for providing long term enteral nutrition. Feeding through PEG tube helps improving the physical growth and general health of the chronically ill patients, with subsequent effect on the family quality of life. The procedure is associated with frequent minor morbidity. Awarness of these complications and the use of preventive strategies can allow the endoscopist to maximize outcomes and to identify complications early.

10. References

Ahmad, I., Mouncher, A., Abdoolah, A., Stenson, R., Wright, J., Daniels, A., Tillett, J., Hawthorne, A. B. & Thomas, G. (2003) Antibiotic prophylaxis for percutaneous endoscopic gastrostomy--a prospective, randomised, double-blind trial. *Aliment Pharmacol Ther,* 18, 209-15.

Anthony, H., Paxton, S., Catto-Smith, A. & Phelan, P. (1999) Physiological and psychosocial contributors to malnutrition in children with cystic fibrosis: review. *Clin Nutr,* 18, 327-35.

Avitsland, T. L., Kristensen, C., Emblem, R., Veenstra, M., Mala, T. & Bjornland, K. (2006) Percutaneous endoscopic gastrostomy in children: a safe technique with major symptom relief and high parental satisfaction. *J Pediatr Gastroenterol Nutr,* 43, 624-8.

Beasley, S. W., Catto-Smith, A. G. & Davidson, P. M. (1995) How to avoid complications during percutaneous endoscopic gastrostomy. *J Pediatr Surg,* 30, 671-3.

Bell, S. C., Elborn, J. S., Campbell, I. A. & Shale, D. J. (1995) Candida albicans infection complicating percutaneous gastrostomy in cystic fibrosis. *Br J Clin Pract,* 49, 109-10.

Belli, D. C., Seidman, E., Bouthillier, L., Weber, A. M., Roy, C. C., Pletincx, M., Beaulieu, M. & Morin, C. L. (1988) Chronic intermittent elemental diet improves growth failure in children with Crohn's disease. *Gastroenterology,* 94, 603-10.

Bellisle, F., Dartois, A. M., Kleinknecht, C. & Broyer, M. (1995) [Alteration of the taste for sugar in renal insufficiency: study in the child]. *Nephrologie,* 16, 203-8.

Berger, S. A. & Zarling, E. J. (1991) Colocutaneous fistula following migration of PEG tube. *Gastrointest Endosc,* 37, 86-8.

Berry, D. P. & Vellacott, K. D. (1992) High jejunal obstruction: a complication of percutaneous endoscopic gastrostomy. *Br J Surg,* 79, 1171.

Borgstein, E. S., Heij, H. A., Beugelaar, J. D., Ekkelkamp, S. & Vos, A. (1994) Risks and benefits of antireflux operations in neurologically impaired children. *Eur J Pediatr,* 153, 248-51.

Bosaeus, I., Daneryd, P., Svanberg, E. & Lundholm, K. (2001) Dietary intake and resting energy expenditure in relation to weight loss in unselected cancer patients. *Int J Cancer,* 93, 380-3.

Bozkurt, M., Tutuncuoglu, S., Serdaroglu, G., Tekgul, H. & Aydogdu, S. (2004) Gastroesophageal reflux in children with cerebral palsy: efficacy of cisapride. *J Child Neurol,* 19, 973-6.

Brant, C. Q., Stanich, P. & Ferrari, A. P., JR. (1999) Improvement of children's nutritional status after enteral feeding by PEG: an interim report. *Gastrointest Endosc,* 50, 183-8.

Brook, I. (1995) Microbiology of gastrostomy site wound infections in children. *J Med Microbiol,* 43, 221-3.

Buchdahl, R. M., Cox, M., Fulleylove, C., Marchant, J. L., Tomkins, A. M., Brueton, M. J. & Warner, J. O. (1988) Increased resting energy expenditure in cystic fibrosis. *J Appl Physiol,* 64, 1810-6.

Buchman, A. L. (2007) Use of percutaneous endoscopic gastrostomy or percutaneous endoscopic jejunostomy in short bowel syndrome. *Gastrointest Endosc Clin N Am,* 17, 787-94.

Cameron, B. H., Blair, G. K., Murphy, J. J., 3rd & Fraser, G. C. (1995) Morbidity in neurologically impaired children after percutaneous endoscopic versus Stamm gastrostomy. *Gastrointest Endosc,* 42, 41-4.

Cosgrove, M. & Jenkins, H. R. (1997) Experience of percutaneous endoscopic gastrostomy in children with Crohn's disease. *Arch Dis Child,* 76, 141-3.

Craig, G. M., Carr, L. J., Cass, H., Hastings, R. P., Lawson, M., Reilly, S., Ryan, M., Townsend, J. & Spitz, L. (2006) Medical, surgical, and health outcomes of gastrostomy feeding. *Dev Med Child Neurol,* 48, 353-60.

Durie, P. R. & Pencharz, P. B. (1992) Cystic fibrosis: nutrition. *Br Med Bull,* 48, 823-46.

Dwyer, K. M., Watts, D. D., Thurber, J. S., Benoit, R. S. & Fakhry, S. M. (2002) Percutaneous endoscopic gastrostomy: the preferred method of elective feeding tube placement in trauma patients. *J Trauma,* 52, 26-32.

Efrati, O., Mei-Zahav, M., Rivilin J., Kerem, E., Blau, H., Barak, A., Bijanover, Y., Augarten, A., Cochavi, B., Yahav, Y. & Modan-Moses, D. (2006) Long term nutritional rehabilitation by gastrostomy in Israeli patients with cystic fibrosis: clinical outcome in advanced pulmonary disease. *J Pediatr Gastroenterol Nutr,* 42, 222-8.

El-Rifai, N., Michaud, L., Mention, K., Guimber, D., Caldari, D., Turck, D. & Gottrand, F. (2004) Persistence of gastrocutaneous fistula after removal of gastrostomy tubes in children: prevalence and associated factors. *Endoscopy,* 36, 700-4.

Farreli, L. D., Karl, S. R., Davis, P. K., Bellinger, M. F. & Ballantine, T. V. (1988) Postoperative necrotizing fasciitis in children. *Pediatrics,* 82, 874-9.

Fonkalsrud, E. W., Ellis, D. G., Shaw, A., Mann, C. M., JR., Black, T. L., Miller, J. P. & Snyder, C. L. (1995) A combined hospital experience with fundoplication and gastric emptying procedure for gastroesophageal reflux in children. *J Am Coll Surg,* 180, 449-55.

Fox, V. L., Abel, S. D., Malas, S., Duggan, C. & Leichtner, A. M. (1997) Complications following percutaneous endoscopic gastrostomy and subsequent catheter replacement in children and young adults. *Gastrointest Endosc,* 45, 64-71.

Furlano, R. I., Sidler, M. & Haack, H. (2008) The push-pull T technique: an easy and safe procedure in children with the buried bumper syndrome. *Nutr Clin Pract,* 23, 655-7.

Galat, S. A., Gerig, K. D., Porter, J. A. & Slezak, F. A. (1990) Management of premature removal of the percutaneous gastrostomy. *Am Surg,* 56, 733-6.

Gangil, A., Patwari, A. K., Bajaj, P., Kashyap, R. & Anand, V. K. (2001) Gastroesophageal reflux disease in children with cerebral palsy. *Indian Pediatr,* 38, 766-70.

Gauderer, M. W. (1991) Percutaneous endoscopic gastrostomy: a 10-year experience with 220 children. *J Pediatr Surg,* 26, 288-92; discussion 292-4.

Gauderer, M. W. (2002) Percutaneous endoscopic gastrostomy and the evolution of contemporary long-term enteral access. *Clin Nutr,* 21, 103-10.

Gisel, E. G., Birnbaum, R. & Schwartz, S. (1998) Feeding impairments in children: diagnosis and effective intervention. *Int J Orofacial Myology,* 24, 27-33.

Giuliano, A., Lewis, F., JR., Hardey, K. & Blaisdell, F. W. (1977) Bacteriology of necrotizing fasciitis. *Am J Surg,* 134, 52-7.

Gottfried, E. B., Plumser, A. B. & Clair, M. R. (1986) Pneumoperitoneum following percutaneous endoscopic gastrostomy. A prospective study. *Gastrointest Endosc,* 32, 397-9.

Hacker, J. F., 3rd & Cattau, E. L., JR. (1987) Conversion of percutaneous endoscopic gastrostomy to a tube colostomy. *South Med J,* 80, 797-8.

Hagelgans, N. A. & Janusz, H. B. (1994) Pediatric skin care issues for the home care nurse: Part 2. *Pediatr Nurs,* 20, 69-74, 76.

Halsey, N. A., Boulos, R., Holt, E., Ruff, A., Brutus, J. R., Kissinger, P., Quinn, T. C., Coberly, J. S., Adrien, M. & Boulos, C. (1990) Transmission of HIV-1 infections from mothers to infants in Haiti. Impact on childhood mortality and malnutrition. The CDS/JHU AIDS Project Team. *JAMA,* 264, 2088-92.

Han-Markey, T. (2000) Nutritional considerations in pediatric oncology. *Semin Oncol Nurs,* 16, 146-51.

Haynes, L., Atherton, D. J., Ade-Ajayi, N., Wheeler, R. & Kiely, E. M. (1996) Gastrostomy and growth in dystrophic epidermolysis bullosa. *Br J Dermatol,* 134, 872-9.

Heikenen, J. B., Werlin, S. L. & Brown, C. W. (1999) Electrogastrography in gastrostomy-tube-fed children. *Dig Dis Sci,* 44, 1293-7.

HEenderson R. A., Saavedra, J. M., Perman, J. A., Hutton, N., Livingston, R. A. & Yolken, R. H. (1994) Effect of enteral tube feeding on growth of children with symptomatic human immunodeficiency virus infection. *J Pediatr Gastroenterol Nutr,* 18, 429-34.

Hillman, K. M. (1982) Pneumoperitoneum--a review. *Crit Care Med,* 10, 476-81.

Hodges, E. G., Morano, J. U. & Nowicki, M. J. (2001) The buried bumper syndrome complicating percutaneous endoscopic gastrostomy in children. *J Pediatr Gastroenterol Nutr,* 33, 326-8.

Hofner, G., Behrens, R., Koch, A., Singer, H. & Hofbeck, M. (2000) Enteral nutritional support by percutaneous endoscopic gastrostomy in children with congenital heart disease. *Pediatr Cardiol,* 21, 341-6.

Hussain, M. & Thambidorai, C. R. (2000) Intussusception as a complication of gastrostomy tube: a case report. *Med J Malaysia,* 55, 271-2.

Iber, F. L., Livak, A. & Patel, M. (1996) Importance of fungus colonization in failure of silicone rubber percutaneous gastrostomy tubes (PEGs). *Dig Dis Sci,* 41, 226-31.

Isch, J. A., Rescorla, F. J., Scherer, L. R., 3rd, West, K. W. & Grosfeld, J. L. (1997) The development of gastroesophageal reflux after percutaneous endoscopic gastrostomy. *J Pediatr Surg,* 32, 321-2; discussion 322-3.

Israel, D. M. & Hassall, E. (1995) Prolonged use of gastrostomy for enteral hyperalimentation in children with Crohn's disease. *Am J Gastroenterol,* 90, 1084-8.

Jafri, N. S., Mahid, S. S., Minor, K. S., Idstein, S. R., Hornung, C. A. & Galandiuk, S. (2007) Meta-analysis: antibiotic prophylaxis to prevent peristomal infection following percutaneous endoscopic gastrostomy. *Aliment Pharmacol Ther,* 25, 647-56.

Kari, J. A., Gonzalez, C., Ledermann, S. E., Shaw, V. & Rees, L. (2000) Outcome and growth of infants with severe chronic renal failure. *Kidney Int,* 57, 1681-7.

Kazi, S., Gunasekaran, T. S., Berman, J. H., Kavin, H. & Kraut, J. R. (1997) Gastric mucosal injuries in children from inflatable low-profile gastrostomy tubes. *J Pediatr Gastroenterol Nutr,* 24, 75-8.

Kealey, W. D., Mccallion, W. A. & Boston, V. E. (1996) Tension pneumoperitoneum: a potentially life-threatening complication of percutaneous endoscopic gastrojejunostomy. *J Pediatr Gastroenterol Nutr,* 22, 334-5.

Khattak, I. U., Kimber, C., Kiely, E. M. & Spitz, L. (1998) Percutaneous endoscopic gastrostomy in paediatric practice: complications and outcome. *J Pediatr Surg,* 33, 67-72.

Kimber, C. P., Khattak, I. U., Kiely, E. M. & Spitz, L. (1998) Peritonitis following percutaneous gastrostomy in children: management guidelines. *Aust N Z J Surg,* 68, 268-70.

Kirschner, B. S., Voinchet, O. & Rosenberg, I. H. (1978) Growth retardation in inflammatory bowel disease. *Gastroenterology,* 75, 504-11.

Klein, S., Heare, B. R. & Soloway, R. D. (1990) The "buried bumper syndrome": a complication of percutaneous endoscopic gastrostomy. *Am J Gastroenterol,* 85, 448-51.

Kobak, G. E., Mcclenathan, D. T. & Schurman, S. J. (2000) Complications of removing percutaneous endoscopic gastrostomy tubes in children. *J Pediatr Gastroenterol Nutr,* 30, 404-7.

Kohler, H., Lang, T. & Behrens, R. (2008) Buried bumper syndrome after percutaneous endoscopic gastrostomy in children and adolescents. *Endoscopy,* 40 Suppl 2, E85-6.

Kraemer, R., Rudenberg A., Hadorn, B. & Rossi, E. (1978) Relative underweight in cystic fibrosis and its prognostic value. *Acta Paediatr Scand,* 67, 33-7.

Lapey, A., Kattwinkel, J., Di Sant'Agnese, P. A. & Laster, L. (1974) Steatorrhea and azotorrhea and their relation to growth and nutrition in adolescents and young adults with cystic fibrosis. *J Pediatr,* 84, 328-34.

Larson, D. E., Burton, D. D., Schroeder, K. W. & Dimagno, E. P. (1987) Percutaneous endoscopic gastrostomy. Indications, success, complications, and mortality in 314 consecutive patients. *Gastroenterology,* 93, 48-52.

Lattuneddu, A., Morgagni, P., Benati, G., Delvecchio, S. & Garcea, D. (2003) Small bowel perforation after incomplete removal of percutaneous endoscopic gastrostomy catheter. *Surg Endosc,* 17, 2028-31.

Lau, G. & Lai, S. H. (2001) Fatal retroperitoneal haemorrhage: an unusual complication of percutaneous endoscopic gastrostomy. *Forensic Sci Int,* 116, 69-75.

Ledermann, S. (2005) When should gastrostomy tubes be removed following successful renal transplantation? *Pediatr Transplant,* 9, 553-4.

Ledermann, S. E., Spitz, L., Moloney, J., Rees, L. & Trompeter, R. S. (2002) Gastrostomy feeding in infants and children on peritoneal dialysis. *Pediatr Nephrol,* 17, 246-50.

Lee, M. P. (1990) Impaction of gastrostomy tube in the abdominal wall. *J Am Geriatr Soc,* 38, 956.

Leitch, C. A. (2000) Growth, nutrition and energy expenditure in pediatric heart failure. *Prog Pediatr Cardiol,* 11, 195-202.

Lowe, J. B., Page, C. P., Schwesinger, W. H., GaskilL, H. V. & Stauffer, J. S. (1997) Percutaneous endoscopic gastrostomy tube placement in a surgical training program. *Am J Surg,* 174, 624-7; discussion 627-8.

Ma, M. M., Semlacher, E. A., Fedorak, R. N., Lalor, E. A., Duerksen, D. R., SherbaniuK, R. W., Chalpelsky, C. E. & Sadowski, D. C. (1995) The buried gastrostomy bumper syndrome: prevention and endoscopic approaches to removal. *Gastrointest Endosc,* 41, 505-8.

Mak, R. H., Cheung, W., Cone, R. D. & Marks, D. L. (2006) Leptin and inflammation-associated cachexia in chronic kidney disease. *Kidney Int,* 69, 794-7.

Marin, O. E., Glassman, M. S., Schoen, B. T. & Caplan, D. B. (1994) Safety and efficacy of percutaneous endoscopic gastrostomy in children. *Am J Gastroenterol,* 89, 357-61.

Matsui, D. M. (1997) Drug compliance in pediatrics. Clinical and research issues. *Pediatr Clin North Am,* 44, 1-14.

Michaud, L., Guimber, D., Carpentier, B., Sfeir, R., Lambilliotte, A., Mazingue, F., Gottrand, F. & Turck, D. (2001) Gastrostomy as a decompression technique in children with chronic gastrointestinal obstruction. *J Pediatr Gastroenterol Nutr,* 32, 82-5.

Milanchi, S. & Allins, A. (2007) Early pneumoperitoneum after percutaneous endoscopic gastrostomy in intensive care patients: sign of possible bowel injury. *Am J Crit Care,* 16, 132-6.

Miller, T. L., Awnetwant, E. L., Evans, S., Morris, V. M., Vazquez, I. M. & McIntosh K. (1995) Gastrostomy tube supplementation for HIV-infected children. *Pediatrics,* 96, 696-702.

Miller, T. L., Evans, S. J., Orav, E. J., Morris, V., McIntosh, K. & Winter, H. S. (1993) Growth and body composition in children infected with the human immunodeficiency virus-1. *Am J Clin Nutr,* 57, 588-92.

Mitchell, I. M., Logan, R. W., Pollock, J. C. & Jamieson, M. P. (1995) Nutritional status of children with congenital heart disease. *Br Heart J,* 73, 277-83.

Mollitt, D. L., Dokler, M. L., Evans, J. S., Jeiven, S. D. & George, D. E. (1998) Complications of retained internal bolster after pediatric percutaneous endoscopic gastrostomy. *J Pediatr Surg,* 33, 271-3.

Morton, R. E., Wheatley, R. & Minford, J. (1999) Respiratory tract infections due to direct and reflux aspiration in children with severe neurodisability. *Dev Med Child Neurol,* 41, 329-34.

Nelson, A. M. (1989) PEG feeding tube migration and erosion into the abdominal wall. *Gastrointest Endosc,* 35, 133.

Oliver, M. R., Heine, R. G., NG, C. H., Volders, E. & Olinsky, A. (2004) Factors affecting clinical outcome in gastrostomy-fed children with cystic fibrosis. *Pediatr Pulmonol,* 37, 324-9.

Palmer, G. M., Frawley, G. P., Heine, R. G. & Oliver, M. R. (2006) Complications associated with endoscopic removal of percutaneous endoscopic gastrostomy (PEG) tubes in children. *J Pediatr Gastroenterol Nutr,* 42, 443-5.

Pashankar, D. & Israel, D. M. (1997) Gastrostomy in children with Crohn's disease. *Arch Dis Child,* 77, 369.

Pedersen, A. M., Kok, K., Petersen, G., Nielsen, O. H., Michaelsen, K. F. & Schmiegelow, K. (1999) Percutaneous endoscopic gastrostomy in children with cancer. *Acta Paediatr,* 88, 849-52.

Pugh, P. & Watson, A. R. (2006) Transition from gastrostomy to oral feeding following renal transplantation. *Adv Perit Dial,* 22, 153-7.

Puntis, J. W., Thwaites, R., Abel, G. & Stringer, M. D. (2000) Children with neurological disorders do not always need fundoplication concomitant with percutaneous endoscopic gastrostomy. *Dev Med Child Neurol,* 42, 97-9.

Ravelli, A. M., Ledermann, S. E., Bisset, W. M., Trompeter, R. S., BarratT, T. M. & Milla, P. J. (1992) Foregut motor function in chronic renal failure. *Arch Dis Child,* 67, 1343-7.

Rees, L. & Shaw, V. (2007) Nutrition in children with CRF and on dialysis. *Pediatr Nephrol,* 22, 1689-702.

Reilly, S. & Skuse, D. (1992) Characteristics and management of feeding problems of young children with cerebral palsy. *Dev Med Child Neurol,* 34, 379-88.

Rempel, G. R., Colwell, S. O. & Nelson, R. P. (1988) Growth in children with cerebral palsy fed via gastrostomy. *Pediatrics,* 82, 857-62.

Ricciardi, E. & Brown, D. (1994) Managing PEG tubes. *Am J Nurs,* 94, 29-31.

Rickard, K. A., Grosfeld, J. L., Coates, T. D., Weetman, R. & Baehner, R. L. (1986) Advances in nutrition care of children with neoplastic diseases: a review of treatment, research, and application. *J Am Diet Assoc,* 86, 1666-76.

Rogers, B., Arvedson, J., Buck, G., Smart, P. & Msall, M. (1994) Characteristics of dysphagia in children with cerebral palsy. *Dysphagia,* 9, 69-73.

Ross, M. N., Haase, G. M., Reiley, T. T. & Meagher, D. P., JR. (1988) The importance of acid reflux patterns in neurologically damaged children detected by four-channel esophageal pH monitoring. *J Pediatr Surg,* 23, 573-6.

Saadeddin, A., Freshwater, D. A., Fisher, N. C. & Jones, B. J. (2005) Antibiotic prophylaxis for percutaneous endoscopic gastrostomy for non-malignant conditions: a double-blind prospective randomized controlled trial. *Aliment Pharmacol Ther,* 22, 565-70.

Sala, A., Pencharz, P. & Barr, R. D. (2004) Children, cancer, and nutrition--A dynamic triangle in review. *Cancer,* 100, 677-87.

Sanders, K. D., Cox, K., Cannon, R., Blanchard, D., Pitcher, J., Papathakis, P., Varella, L. & Maughan, R. (1990) Growth response to enteral feeding by children with cerebral palsy. *JPEN J Parenter Enteral Nutr,* 14, 23-6.

Sanderson, I. R., Udeen, S., Davies, P. S., Savage, M. O. & Walker-Smith, J. A. (1987) Remission induced by an elemental diet in small bowel Crohn's disease. *Arch Dis Child,* 62, 123-7.

Schwartz, H. I., Goldberg, R. I., Barkin, J. S., Phillips, R. S., Land, A. & Hecht, M. (1989) PEG feeding tube migration impaction in the abdominal wall. *Gastrointest Endosc,* 35, 134.

Senac, M. O., JR. & Lee, F. A. (1983) Small-bowel volvulus as a complication of gastrostomy. *Radiology,* 149, 136.

Shallman, R. W., Norfleet, R. G. & Hardache, J. M. (1988) Percutaneous endoscopic gastrostomy feeding tube migration and impaction in the abdominal wall. *Gastrointest Endosc,* 34, 367-8.

Shapiro, B. K., Green, P., Krick, J., Allen, D. & Capute, A. J. (1986) Growth of severely impaired children: neurological versus nutritional factors. *Dev Med Child Neurol,* 28, 729-33.

Shepherd, R., Cooksley, W. G. & Cooke, W. D. (1980) Improved growth and clinical, nutritional, and respiratory changes in response to nutritional therapy in cystic fibrosis. *J Pediatr,* 97, 351-7.

Shingadia, D., Viani, R. M., Yogev, R., Binns, H., Dankner, W. M., Spector, S. A. & CHADWICK, E. G. (2000) Gastrostomy tube insertion for improvement of adherence to highly active antiretroviral therapy in pediatric patients with human immunodeficiency virus. *Pediatrics,* 105, E80.

Siegel, T. R. & Douglass, M. (2004) Perforation of an ileostomy by a retained percutaneous endoscopic gastrostomy (PEG) tube bumper. *Surg Endosc,* 18, 348.

Skolin, I., Hernell, O., Larsson, M. V., Wahlgren, C. & Wahlin, Y. B. (2002) Percutaneous endoscopic gastrostomy in children with malignant disease. *J Pediatr Oncol Nurs,* 19, 154-63.

Smith, D. E., Stevens, M. C. & Booth, I. W. (1991) Malnutrition at diagnosis of malignancy in childhood: common but mostly missed. *Eur J Pediatr,* 150, 318-22.

Sondheimer, J. M. & Morris, B. A. (1979) Gastroesophageal reflux among severely retarded children. *J Pediatr,* 94, 710-4.

Stallings, V. A., Charney, E. B., Davies, J. C. & Cronk, C. E. (1993) Nutrition-related growth failure of children with quadriplegic cerebral palsy. *Dev Med Child Neurol,* 35, 126-38.

Stevenson, R. (2005) Beyond growth: gastrostomy feeding in children with cerebral palsy. *Dev Med Child Neurol,* 47, 76.

Sulaeman, E., Udall, J. N., JR., Brown, R. F., Mannick, E. E., Loe, W. A., Hill, C. B. & Schmidt-Sommerfeld, E. (1998) Gastroesophageal reflux and Nissen fundoplication following percutaneous endoscopic gastrostomy in children. *J Pediatr Gastroenterol Nutr,* 26, 269-73.

Sullivan, P. B. (1992) Gastrostomy and the disabled child. *Dev Med Child Neurol,* 34, 552-5.

Sullivan, P. B. (1999) Gastrostomy feeding in the disabled child: when is an antireflux procedure required? *Arch Dis Child,* 81, 463-4.

Sullivan, P. B., Juszczak, E., Bachlet, A. M., Lambert, B., Vernon-Roberts, A., Grant, H. W., Eltumi, M., Mclean, L., Alder, N. & Thomas, A. G. (2005) Gastrostomy tube feeding in children with cerebral palsy: a prospective, longitudinal study. *Dev Med Child Neurol,* 47, 77-85.

Sullivan, P. B., Juszczak, E., Bachlet, A. M., Thomas, A. G., Lambert, B., Vernon-Roberts, A., Grant, H. W., Eltumi, M., Alder, N. & Jenkinson, C. (2004) Impact of gastrostomy tube feeding on the quality of life of carers of children with cerebral palsy. *Dev Med Child Neurol,* 46, 796-800.

Sullivan, P. B., Lambert, B., Rose, M., Ford-Adams, M., Johnson, A. & Griffiths, P. (2000) Prevalence and severity of feeding and nutritional problems in children with neurological impairment: Oxford Feeding Study. *Dev Med Child Neurol,* 42, 674-80.

Sy, K., Dipchand, A., Atenafu, E., Chait, P., Bannister, L., Temple, M., John, P., Connolly, B. & Amaral, J. G. (2008) Safety and effectiveness of radiologic percutaneous gastrostomy and gastro jejunostomy in children with cardiac disease. *AJR Am J Roentgenol,* 191, 1169-74.

Tawfik, R., Dickson, A., Clarke, M. & Thomas, A. G. (1997) Caregivers' perceptions following gastrostomy in severely disabled children with feeding problems. *Dev Med Child Neurol,* 39, 746-51.

Taylor, L. A., Weiner, T., Lacey, S. R. & Azizkhan, R. G. (1994) Chronic lung disease is the leading risk factor correlating with the failure (wrap disruption) of antireflux procedures in children. *J Pediatr Surg,* 29, 161-4; discussion 164-6.

Temple, M. E., Koranyi, K. I. & Nahata, M. C. (2001) Gastrostomy tube placement in nonadherent HIV-infected children. *Ann Pharmacother,* 35, 414-8.

Tisdale, M. J. (1997) Cancer cachexia: metabolic alterations and clinical manifestations. *Nutrition,* 13, 1-7.

Truby, H., Cowlishaw, P., O'Neill C. & Waineright, C. (2009) The long term efficacy of gastrostomy feeding in children with cystic fibrosis on anthropometric markers of nutritonal status and pulmonary function. *Open Respir Med J,* 3, 112-5.

Van Biervliet, S., De Waele, K., Van Winckel, M. & Robberecht, E. (2004) Percutaneous endoscopic gastrostomy in cystic fibrosis: patient acceptance and effect of overnight tube feeding on nutritional status. *Acta Gastroenterol Belg,* 67, 241-4.

Van Eys, J. (1979) Malnutrition in children with cancer: incidence and consequence. *Cancer,* 43, 2030-5.

Von Schnakenburg, C., Feneberg, R., Plank, C., Zimmering, M., Arbeiter, K., Bald, M., Fehrenbach, H., Griebel, M., Licht, C., Konrad, M., Timmermann, K. & Kemper, M. J. (2006) Percutaneous endoscopic gastrostomy in children on peritoneal dialysis. *Perit Dial Int,* 26, 69-77.

Watson, A. R. (2006) Gastrostomy feeding in children on chronic peritoneal dialysis. *Perit Dial Int,* 26, 41-2.

Waxman, I., Al-Kawas, F. H., Bass, B. & Glouderman, M. (1991) PEG ileus. A new cause of small bowel obstruction. *Dig Dis Sci,* 36, 251-4.

Weiss, B., Fradkin, A., Ben-Akun, M., Avigad, I., Ben-Shlush, A. & Jonas, A. (1999) Upper gastrointestinal bleeding due to gastric ulcers in children with gastrostomy tubes. *J Clin Gastroenterol,* 29, 48-50.

Wiggins, T. F., Kaplan, R. & Delegge, M. H. (2007) Acute hemorrhage following transhepatic PEG tube placement. *Dig Dis Sci,* 52, 167-9.

Wojyowycz, M. M., Arata, J. A., JR., Micklos, T. J. & Miller, F. J., JR. (1988) CT findings after uncomplicated percutaneous gastrostomy. *AJR Am J Roentgenol,* 151, 307-9.

Yaseen, M., Steele, M. I. & Grunow, J. E. (1996) Nonendoscopic removal of percutaneous endoscopic gastrostomy tubes: morbidity and mortality in children. *Gastrointest Endosc,* 44, 235-8.

Part 2

Indications of Gastrostomy in the Adults

4

Percutaneous Endoscopic Gastrostomy in Neurological Patients

David T. Burke and Andrew I. Geller
Department of Physical Medicine and Rehabilitation, Emory University, Atlanta, Georgia USA

1. Introduction

Patients with neurologic dysfunction are at increased risk for malnutrition due to a combination of cognitive, behavioral and mechanical problems. Cohort studies have shown that 20-50% of hospital patients are malnourished (McWhirter & Pennington, 1994; Norman et al., 2008; Kurien et al., 2010), and 20-40% of critically ill patients show evidence of protein-energy malnutrition (Ziegler, 2009). Access for supplemental nutrition may be considered to meet the nutritional needs of any patient with a functional gastrointestinal tract who is unable to safely swallow (Kulick & Deen, 2011; McClave et al., 2009). The primary aim of enteral tube feeding is to avoid further loss of body weight, to correct significant nutritional deficiencies, to rehydrate the patient, to promote growth in children with growth retardation, and to stop the related deterioration of the quality of life of the patient due to inadequate oral nutrition intake (Loser et al., 2005). A variety of enteric feeding tube options exist, including endoscopically-placed nasogastric feeding tubes, percutaneous endoscopic gastrostomy (PEG), radiologically inserted gastrostomy (RIG), and per-oral image guided gastrostomy (PIG) (Laasch et al., 2003; Hoffer et al., 1999; Preshaw, 1981; Tao & Gillies, 1983; Wills & Oglesby, 1983; Gauderer et al., 1980). The endoscopic access routes have been more popular than radiologic routes, which despite being quite effective have been reserved as a PEG alternative in cases deemed too risky or difficult for the passage of an endoscope (de Baere et al., 1999; Galaski et al., 2009; Loser et al., 2005; Ozmen & Akhan, 2002). Enteral access can also be obtained surgically, but this has become much less frequent since the advent of these less-invasive techniques (Duszak & Mabry, 2003; Sleisenger et al., 2010). In cases where endoscopic access is not obtained, technical considerations and/or local availability play a role in determining whether a patient receives a radiological or surgical gastrostomy (Kurien et al., 2010; Leeds et al., 2010; Ljungdahl & Sundbom, 2006).

2. Techniques commonly employed in early feeding

The incidence of malnutrition worsens over time in patients who require prolonged hospitalization. Malnutrition is associated with increased morbidity and mortality in hospitalized patients; protein-calorie malnutrition is associated with skeletal muscle weakness, an increased rate of hospital-acquired infection, impaired wound healing, and prolonged recovery time. The relationship between malnutrition and adverse clinical outcomes is complex. Patients who are more difficult to feed are more critically ill and at higher risk for death and complications. Commonly-employed techniques for early feeding to address nutritional deficiency include parenteral, nasogastric and nasoenteric feeding.

2.1 Parenteral access

In most cases enteral feeding is a viable option early during the course of hospitalization. Although early enteral nutrition has been shown to be associated with a significantly lower incidence of infections and a reduced length of hospital stay (Marik & Zaloga, 2001), enteral feeding is not always possible. In such cases, parenteral hydration and nutrition may be the only option to maintain healthy levels of fluid and nutrition. Studies suggest that in these instances patients with moderate-to-severe protein-energy malnutrition may benefit from parenteral nutrition (Heyland et al., 1998). Published guidelines suggest that when enteral feeding is not possible, parenteral nutrition should be initiated within 3-7 days; among such patients who have protein-energy malnutrition at the time of admission to the intensive care unit, the American Clinical Practice Guidelines suggest that parenteral nutrition should be initiated without delay (Ziegler, 2009).

This is not an option without inherent risks. A meta-analysis of well-designed intention-to-treat trials comparing enteral nutrition with parenteral nutrition in critically ill patients (with each study enrolling fewer than 200 patients) showed a significant reduction in mortality among patients receiving parenteral nutrition (Simpson & Doig, 2005). The risk of infection was significantly increased with parenteral nutrition. A systematic review of 13 randomized clinical trials involving critically ill adults showed a significant reduction in infectious complications with enteral nutrition, as compared with parenteral nutrition (Gramlich et al., 2004). In general, a catheter that is inserted for parenteral nutrition should not be used for any other purpose, such as phlebotomy or the administration of medications; and particular care must be taken to maintain the catheter and the percutaneous entry site with appropriate sterile access and dressing techniques (Ziegler, 2009; American Society for Parenteral and Enteral Nutrition, 2002; Mirtallo et al., 2004). The estimated daily cost of standard central venous parenteral nutrition is approximately $60 to $90, depending on additives (e.g., supplemental micronutrients). Personnel costs for monitoring by nutritional-support health professionals and for preparation of parenteral nutrition by pharmacists is approximately $20 per day, with additional minor costs for intravenous tubing, nursing time. Central-vein parenteral nutrition may also be associated with mechanical, metabolic, and infectious complications (American Society for Parenteral and Enteral Nutrition, 2002; Ziegler, 2009).

2.2 Nasogastric access

Nasogastric tube (NG) feeding is the most common and oldest form of interventional feeding. Nasogastric tubes have the advantage of being simple to insert but are often poorly tolerated by the patient, and are difficult to maintain in position. They have a significant associated risk of aspiration (Ciocon et al., 1988), and carry a high risk for accidental displacement (Keohane et al., 1986; Payne-James & Silk, 1988).

The benefits of placing a nasogastric tube include the fact that little skill is required for tube placement and it enables early commencement of enteral feeding. This maintains intestinal function. The ability to use the tube for bolus feedings has the added advantage of being more physiologic than is continuous feeding. Manual placement of a nasogastric tube at the bedside, without guidance, is often done without complications. Verification of the placement of the tube was once thought to be sufficiently accomplished by auscultation, listening for a gastric bubble as air is forced into the tube. Extraction of gastric contents is another such verification method: measuring pH of the gastric contents could allow for verification of the fluid extracted as that from the stomach, though in practice this is rarely done. Despite its simplicity, however, this method can result insignificant and potentially lethal complications. These include misplacement, mucosal injury with bleeding and/or esophageal, gastric, or intestinal perforation. These complications require immediate treatment.

Enteral feeding can usually be continued after misplacement or bleeding. With perforation, however, alternative feeding such as Total Parenteral Nutrition (TPN), along with antibiotics and bowel rest, are undertaken. It is common for the nasogastric tube not to be inserted far enough and to be left in the distal esophagus or, in the extreme situation, placed in the trachea or bronchial tree rather than passed into the stomach. These placements will increase the risk of aspiration. To ensure correct placement in the stomach, at least 50 cm of the tube should b. While placement can be initially assessed by the insufflation of 50 mL of air—which should be easily audible by auscultation (with bubbling) in the epigastrium—confirmation of correct placement should be sought by radiography before feeding commences. Correct placement is confirmed when the shadow of the tube is detected below the level of the diaphragm.

The decision to move from a nasogastric tube to a gastrostomy tube is based on a number of factors including the length of time that is being considered for the enteral feeding. Often when initially placed, it is not clear how long will be the need for the NG feeding. What is initially placed as a very short term measure may, due to complications with treatment, evolve into a more chronic situation. The majority of patients requiring nutritional support will need it for less than one month, and nasogastric tube feeding is by far the most commonly used route of access. Fine bore nasogastric tubes have reduced the incidence of complications, such as rhinitis, esophageal reflux, strictures and esophagitis that were associated with the large bore Ryle's tube (Pearce & Duncan, 2002).

2.3 Nasoenteric access

Nasoenteric tube placement is more invasive than the corresponding nasogastric procedure and, therefore, carries a greater risk of mucosal injury if the tube is placed manually. As the control of delivery of fluid by the stomach is bypassed, nasoenteric feeds should be given as a constant infusion and not in bolus form. Furthermore, since the stomach is bypassed, bacterial suppression by gastric acid is lost and a sterile feed must be given via a 'closed' system.

The complications of nasoenteral feeding tubes have become less common since the introduction of fine bore nasoenteral feeding tubes in the 1970s. These tubes are easier to pass, more flexible and are less likely to cause erosions, esophagitis, or strictures. Local complications are common, however, with patients noting discomfort when the tubes are passed, and with tube maintenance as the securing devices are manipulated. This is again dependent largely on the tube's diameter, softness and type of tip. As in other methods of tube access, detection of correct placement is not an insignificant concern. Patients most at risk from misplacement of nasogastric tubes include those on ventilators, those who have altered level of consciousness and/or those with neuromuscular abnormalities, such as reduced gag, swallow, and cough reflexes.

Other complications of nasoenteral access include the development of tracheo-esophageal fistula, which may develop when large-bore nasoenteric tubes are used. Commonly, nasoenteric tubes become displaced, particularly in the critically ill and/or those who have altered levels of consciousness.

Placing nasoenteral feeding tubes postpylorically can be difficult; spontaneous transpyloric passage of standard feeding tubes after 24 hours is only in the order of 30% and does not seem to be affected by tip profile or addition of a weight to the tip of the feeding tube (Pearce & Duncan, 2002).

3. Techniques commonly employed for long-term feeding

As a result of some of the difficulties encountered with nasogastric and nasoenteric feeding tubes, alternative routes of tube feeding have been developed, some of which have proven useful for long term feeding (Pearce & Duncan, 2002). Tube enterostomies can be placed using surgical, endoscopic, or radiological methods into the gastrointestinal tract.

3.1 Percutaneous endoscopic gastrostomy

First described in 1980, PEG has become the most commonly-employed method of enteral access, due to its relative ease of deployment in most patients and overall tolerability. PEG placement is a common indication for endoscopy of the upper gastrointestinal tract (Park et al., 2011; Srinivasan et al., 2009), and is now much more widely used than surgical or radiological insertion. Rates of PEG insertion have risen in recent years: in 1989, 15,000 PEG tubes were placed; in 1995, 121,000 PEG tubes were placed, and in 2000, more than 216,000 tubes were inserted for feeding (Delegge, 2008; Grant et al., 1998; Roche, 2003; Duszak & Mabry, 2003). The greatest increase in feeding tube placement has occurred in those 75 years of age and older (Freeman et al., 2010; Lewis et al., 2004). Various treatment guidelines have been developed to assist clinicians in navigating the clinical and ethical issues informing the decision to place a PEG (Ritchie et al., 2007; Greff, 1999; Loser et al., 2005; Maillet et al., 2002; Niv & Abuksis, 2003; Rosner, 1997).

PEG is commonly used in patients with neurologic dysfunction who have intact cognition and/or a high likelihood to maintain their current baseline, or recover their premorbid neurologic function (DeLegge et al., 2005; Gauderer et al., 1980). A recent meta-analysis found that PEG carries a lower risk of intervention failure when compared with use of nasogastric (NG) tube, although no significant difference in mortality rates between comparison groups, or pneumonia irrespective of underlying disease was found (Gomes et al., 2010). When compared with NG access, PEG has been shown to be a more reliable enteral access tube, allowing patients to receive more calories daily because of a reduction in tube dysfunction (Park et al., 1992; Sleisenger et al., 2010). However, the unproven efficacy of enteral nutrition in prolonging survival and improving quality of life in many clinical settings, and the potential for multiple complications have tempered the "enthusiasm" for performing this procedure for nutritional support in many clinical situations (Potack & Chokhavatia, 2008); nevertheless, gastrostomy feeding has the potential to reduce mortality, length of hospital stay, and complications in carefully selected patients who are likely to be or later become nutritionally depleted for longer than four to six weeks (Green, 1999; Kurien et al., 2010; Wicks et al., 1992).

The gastrostomy tube can be placed via a "pull" (Ponsky-Gauderer) technique, be pushed into place by a "push" (Sacks-Vine) method, or secured via the "introducer" (Russell) procedure, where the stomach is be directly punctured and a Foley catheter placed over a guidewire. A wide variety of commercial PEG systems are available. The tube diameters commonly used range from 6 mm to 8 mm. In general, small-diameter tubes should be avoided in patients with poor gastric emptying who require intragastric administration of medication. If a PEG with jejunal extension is required, such as for patients with gastroparesis, a wide (for example, 8 mm diameter) tube is required that can be cannulated with a narrow (for example, 5.3 mm diameter) jejunal tube (O'Keefe, 2009).

3.1.1 Indications for percutaneous endoscopic gastrostomy

Placement of a PEG tube should be considered for patients who continue to require enteral feeding beyond 4 weeks; it is also indicated as first-line intervention in conditions where enteral feeding is expected to be required for longer than 2–4 weeks (O'Keefe, 2009). Neurogenic indications for gastrostomy include dysphagia from a variety of causes, including stroke, brain injury, cerebral palsy, brain tumors, HIV encephalopathy, neonatal encephalopathy, and neurodegenerative syndromes; non-neurological indications include such conditions as head and neck cancer, surgery to the mouth and throat, aspiration, Crohn's disease, severe burns, and decompression of the stomach in obstructing intra-abdominal malignancy (Buchholz, 1994; Laasch et al., 2003; Nishiwaki et al., 2009; El-Matary, 2008; Naik et al., 2009; Park et al., 2011). The most common indication for PEG in children and adults is neurogenic dysphagia (El-Matary, 2008; Miller et al., 1989; Nicholson et al., 2000; Friedman et al., 2004; Srivastava et al., 2005). Enteral access can also facilitate the delivery of medications in patients whose illness limits their ability to take them by mouth (Phillips & Nay, 2008; El-Matary, 2008; Loser et al., 2005); and it can also facilitate hydration in these patients (Sleisenger et al., 2010).

Neurogenic dysphagia secondary to *stroke* is the most common cause for PEG insertion in adults (James et al., 1998; James et al., 2005; Rimon et al., 2005; Gencosmanoglu, 2004); dysphagia occurs in around 40% of patients at the time of diagnosis, with up to 10% of stroke patients suffering long-term dysphagia (Barer, 1989; Gordon et al., 1987; Kidd et al., 1995; Laasch et al., 2003; O'Neill, 2000; Smithard et al., 1996). Early feeding (within the first week) via PEG is no longer recommended in the most recent guidelines for management of acute stroke, as it has not been shown to improve long-term survival, complication rates or length of hospitalization (Koretz et al., 2007; Kulick & Deen, 2011). More recent guidelines recommend the early initiation of NG tube feeds for dysphagic patients with acute ischemic stroke (within 48 hours), and not placing PEG within the first two weeks (Ringleb et al., 2008). Others have recommended continuing the NG feeds for the first month in patients whose swallow function does not recover (Hill, 2008).

Patients with hypertensive *intracerebral hemorrhage* may benefit from early enteral nutrition based on observational data (Lee et al., 2010); however, no randomized data exist. Data is similarly lacking for the use of PEG in dysphagic patients with *Parkinson's disease* (Deane et al., 2001).

A recent meta-analysis of nutritional support in *head-injured* patients concluded that, while data are lacking, early feeding may be associated with a trend toward better outcomes in terms of survival and disability (Perel et al., 2006).

Amyotrophic Lateral Sclerosis (ALS) is another condition where PEG is routinely employed (James et al., 1998; James et al., 2005; Rimon et al., 2005; Mitsumoto et al., 2003). In addition to progressive issues with dysphagia, ALS patients have increased energy needs, and it has been suggested that PEG can play an important role in preventing additional muscle loss (Desport et al., 1999; Spataro et al., 2011; Vaisman et al., 2009). Recent guidelines recommend ALS patients receive PEG when oral intake is limited and body weight begins to decline (Andersen et al., 2007; Radunovic et al., 2007; Spataro et al., 2011). Some have recommended PEG be placed for weight loss of more than 10% over baseline and before forced vital capacity (FVC) falls below 50%; however, safe PEG insertion has been documented in patients with FVC below 50% (Gregory et al., 2002; Spataro et al., 2011). Limited data from non-randomized studies suggest a survival advantage and improved nutrition with enteral feeding (Katzberg & Benatar, 2011; Chio et al., 1999; Mazzini et al., 1995; Spataro et al., 2011). No randomized controlled trials exist.

Multiple sclerosis (MS) is also associated with progressive dysphagia prompting the use of PEG; small case reports have demonstrated an improvement in comorbid disease states, such as pressure ulcer healing, in patients with MS and dysphagia who receive tube feedings (Annoni et al., 1998; Sleisenger et al., 2010).

More than 36,000 older patients with *dementia* receive a PEG tube each year (Gillick, 2000; Sleisenger et al., 2010). PEG placement in elderly patients with dementia is controversial (Palecek et al., 2010; Delegge, 2009; Garrow et al., 2007; Gillick, 2000; Cervo et al., 2006; Chernoff, 2006). No randomized controlled trials exist in this patient population, and observational studies do not show any evidence of increased survival with PEG; nor was there any reduction in pressure ulcers, improvement in quality of life, function behavior or psychiatric symptoms of dementia (Sampson et al., 2009). However, while earlier data suggested worse clinical outcomes in patients with dementia or significant cognitive impairment who received PEG, more recent data suggests outcomes in these populations are no different than in other patient populations receiving PEG (Freeman et al., 2010; Delegge, 2008; Higaki et al., 2008; Gaines et al., 2009). As in other patient populations, the decision to insert a PEG tube in an elderly demented patient should always be made on an individual basis (National Collaborating Centre for Acute Care, 2006; Kurien et al., 2010; Rabeneck et al., 1997).

In children and adults with *intellectual disability/mental retardation*, feeding via PEG has been shown to improve nutritional status and quality of life in certain patients (Loser et al., 2005; Mathus-Vliegen et al., 2001) but not others (Lee & MacPherson, 2010); no randomized studies have been performed.

3.1.2 Complications of percutaneous endoscopic gastrostomy

Despite its strong safety record, PEG tube placement can be associated with an overall complication rate of 4.9–50% (Amann et al., 1997; Fröhlich et al., 2010). Complications are more likely to occur in elderly patients with comorbid illness, particularly those with an infectious process or who have a history of aspiration (Naik et al., 2009); it is therefore important to recognize that some patients are too frail for the sedation necessary for the endoscopy, particularly those patients with severe respiratory disease (Nicholson et al., 2000). Potential risk factors for complications in younger patients include age less than 1 year, mental retardation, scoliosis, constipation, hepatomegaly, previous upper abdominal surgery, presence of ventriculoperitoneal shunt, peritoneal dialysis and coagulopathy (Fröhlich et al., 2010; Vervloessem et al., 2009; von Schnakenburg et al., 2006).

Inadequate transillumination is considered the primary absolute contraindication for PEG placement because this indicates the inability to oppose the anterior gastric wall to the abdominal wall; this could result from organomegaly, severe ascites or an interposed colon (Nicholson et al., 2000). An absolute containdication to PEG placement is the inability to bring the anterior gastric wall in apposition to the abdominal wall. Prior gastric resection, ascites, hepatomegaly and obesity are some conditions which may impede gastric transillumination and subsequent PEG placement. Percutaneous endoscopic gastrostomy feeding should not be used when gastrointestinal obstruction is present. Relative contraindications to PEG include neoplastic, inflammatory and infiltrative diseases of the gastric and abdominal walls (Nicholson et al., 2000).

Pneumoperitoneum can be rather common among those that receive a PEG. This can occur when air escapes into the peritoneal cavity during the puncture of the abdominal wall and the stomach. In much of medical practice the detection of or air within the peritoneal cavity frequently indicates a perforated abdominal viscus that requires emergent surgical management. On radiograph, pneumoperitoneum appears as a characteristic radiolucency seen below the diaphragm on chest radiograph or in a superiorly dependent location on abdominal radiograph; in the appropriate clinical setting, the radiographic presence of intraperitoneal air often is believed to be a diagnostic finding. In fact, pneumoperitoneum reflects visceral perforation in 85% to 95% of all occurrences. In 5% to 15% of cases, however, pneumoperitoneum does not reflect perforation and results from another source that does not require emergency surgery. In a recent review, the most common abdominal etiology of non-surgical peritoneum (NSP) was retained postoperative air (prevalence 25% to 60%). NSP occurred frequently after peritoneal dialysis catheter placement (prevalence 10% to 34%) and after gastrointestinal endoscopic procedures (prevalence 0.3% to 25%, varying by procedure). The most common thoracic causes included mechanical ventilation, cardiopulmonary resuscitation, and pneumothorax. Clinicians should maintain a high index of suspicion for nonsurgical causes of pneumoperitoneum and should recognize that conservative management may be indicated in many cases (Mularski et al., 2000). In one study of patients undergoing PEG placement, of the 65 patients who underwent PEG placement, 13 developed a pneumoperitoneum on the initial chest radiograph; 10 of the 13 patients experienced complete resolution of pneumoperitoneum at 72 hours, and in 3 patients, the free air persisted but was of no clinical significance (Wiesen et al., 2006). Wiesen et al. conclude that pneumoperitoneum following PEG is of no clinical significance and hence, does not warrant any further intervention (Garcia-Bueno et al., 1998; Wiesen et al., 2006).

Replacement is sometimes required if a PEG is inadvertently removed; premature removal of PEG tubes by either the patient or healthcare staff occurs in 2% of patients and can lead to significant complications if not promptly recognized and appropriately treated (Galat et al., 1990; Larson et al., 1987; Marshall et al., 1994; Orlando Regional Medical Center Department of Surgical Education, 2009). Agitated or delirious patients who inadvertently pull out their PEG tube often can be successfully managed with nasogastric suction and PEG replacement (Galat et al., 1990; Marshall et al., 1994). A Foley catheter can be inserted through the tract and feeding restarted until the PEG is replaced either endoscopically with a standard PEG tube or non-endoscopically with a button gastrostomy. Anecdotally, the PEG tract closes in 24–48 hours when the patient is treated with bowel rest with or without nasogastric suction. Subsequent placement of a PEG tube in a new site is often successful. Signs of peritonitis mandate treatment with antibiotics and a surgical consultation. If a PEG tube is inadvertently removed from a mature tract (> 3–4 weeks old), a Foley catheter can be inserted to maintain tract patency, but this should not be attempted if the PEG tract is immature. Burke et al. have evaluated the use of an air contrast insufflation through a recently replaced gastrostomy tube as a quick and cost-effective method for confirming appropriate positioning. Following an initial case report, the authors subsequently reported their experience with gastrostomy tube confirmation using 240 mL of room air instilled into the stomach, with before and after radiographs. Twenty-nine gastrostomy tubes were replaced using air insufflation and 19 tubes using water-soluble contrast followed by fluoroscopy. At two weeks post-procedure, the authors found no difference between the two techniques in terms of complications or mis-positioned tubes (Burke et al., 2006; Burke et al., 2005; Burke & Hoaglin, 2007; Orlando Regional Medical Center Department of Surgical Education, 2009).

Peritonitis is a feared complication of PEG that often carries a high mortality rate. Intraperitoneal leakage of gastric contents, wound dehiscence, and delayed stoma closure can cause peritonitis (Pearce et al., 2000). Peritonitis complicates up to 2.3% of procedures in large series (Luman et al., 2001). We have previously described the case of a 33-year-old brain-injured patient whose PEG insertion was complicated by inadvertent malpositioning and subsequent infection; after initially being placed through the liver, the PEG tube migrated out several weeks later, resulting in intra-abdominal feed collection, peri-hepatic abscess formation, and peritonitis (Burke & Geller, 2009). Other such cases have been recorded with one large series reporting this in 2.3% of the cases (Luman et al., 2001).

Hemorrhage occurs in up to 2.5% of PEG placements (Larson et al., 1987; Schapiro & Edmundowicz, 1996). During the procedure hemorrhage may be caused by puncture of gastric wall vessels; the most common cause of hemorrhage post-PEG is due to the ulceration of the gastric mucosa underneath the internal bumper when applied in very tight approximation to the mucosa (Potack & Chokhavatia, 2008). Post-PEG hemorrhage is managed similar to other episodes of upper gastrointestinal bleeding. Diagnostic upper endoscopy is often performed. If endoscopy does not reveal a bleeding source, it is useful to loosen the external bolster on the PEG tube to free it from the gastric mucosa and evaluate for underlying ulceration (Cappell & Abdullah, 2000).

Visceral perforation is also a concern in PEG placement. As concerns the small intestine, normally the greater omentum restricts the small bowel from positioning in the upper abdomen; in children with prior abdominal surgery, however, adhesions could displace the small bowel in front of the liver (Fröhlich et al., 2010; Wilson et al., 1990). Small bowel volvulus around the PEG and subsequent obstruction has also been reported (Alawadhi et al., 1991; Al-Homaidhi & Tolia, 2001; Hoffer et al., 1999). Additionally, loosening of the external bolster can allow migration of the internal bumper through the pylorus into the small bowel, mimicking small bowel obstruction (Hoffer et al., 1999; Mollitt et al., 1998; Schrag et al., 2007).

Wound Infection is a common occurrence, with local infection found to occur in up to 23% of cases (Lee et al., 2002). The majority of infections (>70%) are minor (Gossner et al., 1999). Trials of use of prophylactic systemic antibiotics have demonstrated significant reductions in the rate of these infections, while attempts to use topical antibiotics at the peristomal site have been met with much less success. As many patients with PEG tube placement are hospitalized, there is a risk for nosocomial colonization that complicates this use of antibiotics.

Excessive leakage at the peristomal site is one of the more commonly encountered complications of PEG placement, and has been reported in 1-2% of the cases (Lin et al., 2001). It can result from mechanical factors such as side torsion on the tube with ulceration on one side of the tract and absence of an external bolster (McClave & Chang, 2003). Side torsion with ulceration in the tract may require stabilization of the PEG tube with a commercial clamping device that prevents side-to-side motion. If there is increased granulation tissue around the peristomal site, this may be addressed with topical silver nitrate.

Colon perforation is another complication of PEG insertion. The transverse colon is apposed to the greater curvature of the stomach; and if the stomach is not well insufflated during placement of the PEG tube, the colon may not be completely displaced out of the field, thus leading to puncture by the gastrostomy tube (Hogan et al., 1986). One such example is illustrated in Figures 1, 2 and 3. This complication is seen more frequently in pediatric populations, where it occurs at a rate of 2%-3.5% (Khattak et al., 1998). The early presentation of this complication is that of peritonitis or large bowel obstruction, although many patients present months later with partial large bowel obstruction or diarrhea due to leakage of feedings into the colon (Hogan et al., 1986). Intractable diarrhea has been described as a possible presenting sign of PEG placement through the transverse colon (Burke & Carayannopoulos, 2005).

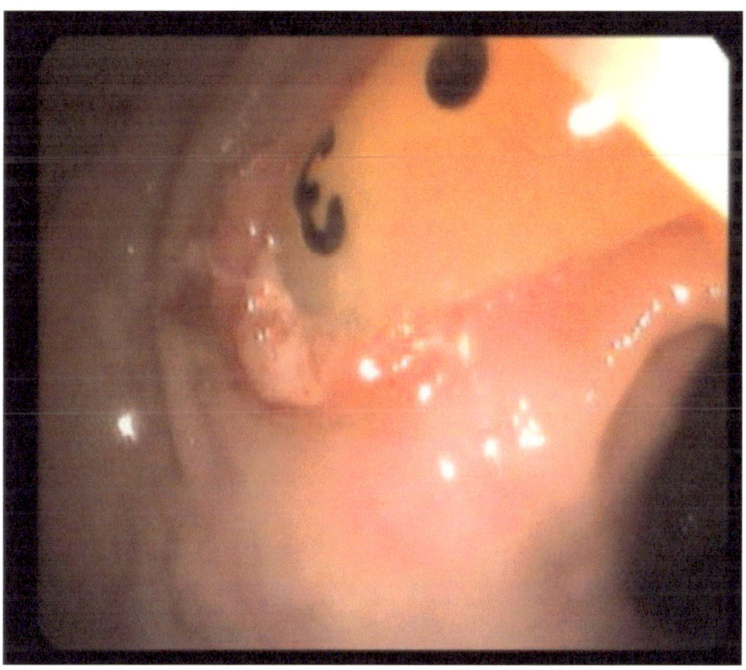

Fig. 1. PEG tube exiting transverse colon

Diagnosis of colon perforation is confirmed by barium enema examination, colonoscopy, or CT scan. Patients who do not manifest signs of obstruction or peritonitis can be managed by tube removal. In most cases, the fistula will close and a second gastrostomy can be performed (Hogan et al., 1986; Potack & Chokhavatia, 2008; Schapiro & Edmundowicz,

1996). If obstruction or peritonitis is present or the fistula does not close despite PEG removal, operative takedown of the fistula is necessary (Cappell & Abdullah, 2000; Patwardhan et al., 2004; Potack & Chokhavatia, 2008; Schapiro & Edmundowicz, 1996). Anecdotal reports support the practice of using a fluid-filled syringe attached to the finder needle during PEG placement for reducing the risk of colonic perforation. Aspiration of air bubbles prior to visualizing the needle in the stomach suggests the presence of interposed bowel between the abdominal wall and stomach (Potack & Chokhavatia, 2008). Friedmann et al. identified 6 hospitalized patients who had misplacement of a PEG into the colon, and a review of the English literature revealed another 22 adult cases with this complication (Friedmann et al., 2007). Of the total 28 cases, 8 had previous abdominal pathology. Seventeen patients developed symptoms after tube replacement, whereas in 11 the tube had not been changed. Fourteen had diarrhea, 11 presented with fecal discharge in or around the tube, and 3 were asymptomatic. Thirteen showed colocutaneous fistula without residual connection to the stomach. Ten patients were treated surgically and 14 conservatively by removal of the tube. One patient had colonoscopic clipping of the fistula. Clinicians should therefore suspect misplacement of the tube into the colon when there is recurrent severe diarrhea of undigested food or fecal content in the tube, particularly after tube replacement; and treatment may be conservative in most cases (Friedmann et al., 2007).

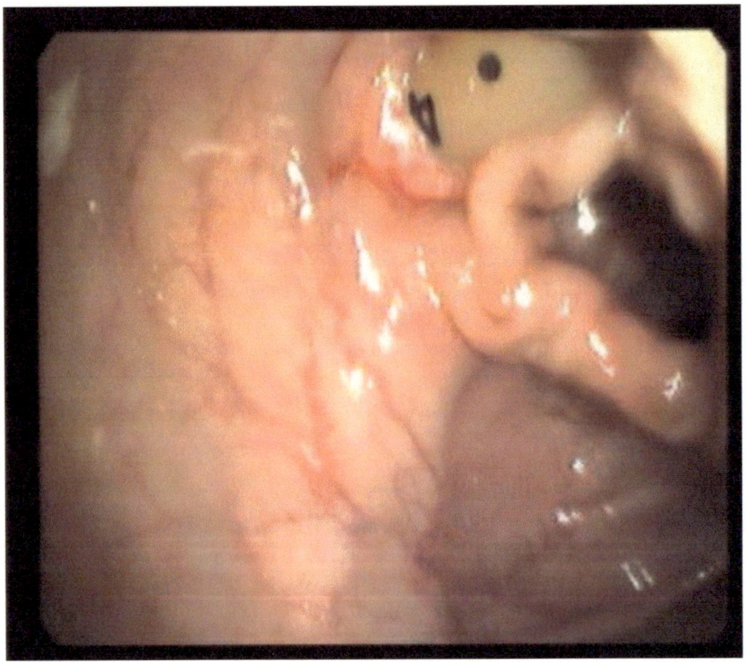

Fig. 2. PEG tube entering transverse colon

Buried bumper syndrome is defined as migration of the PEG tube into the gastric wall and the subsequent epithelization of the ulcer site (Safadi et al., 1998). Buried bumper syndrome often occurs months to years after PEG placement (median duration was 35 months after PEG placement) as the patient develops abdominal pain; difficulty feeding or flushing the tube; and the inability to advance, withdraw, or rotate the tube (Horbach et al., 2007). Buried bumper is thought to arise from excessive traction on the tube causing it to erode into the gastric wall. The incidence of this complication has lessened with newer tube designs which utilize a softer internal bumper (Schapiro & Edmundowicz, 1996). Treatment involves removing the tube (which may require upper endoscopy), allowing the tract to close while an alternative method of feeding is established, and then placing a new PEG tube in a different location (Horbach et al., 2007).

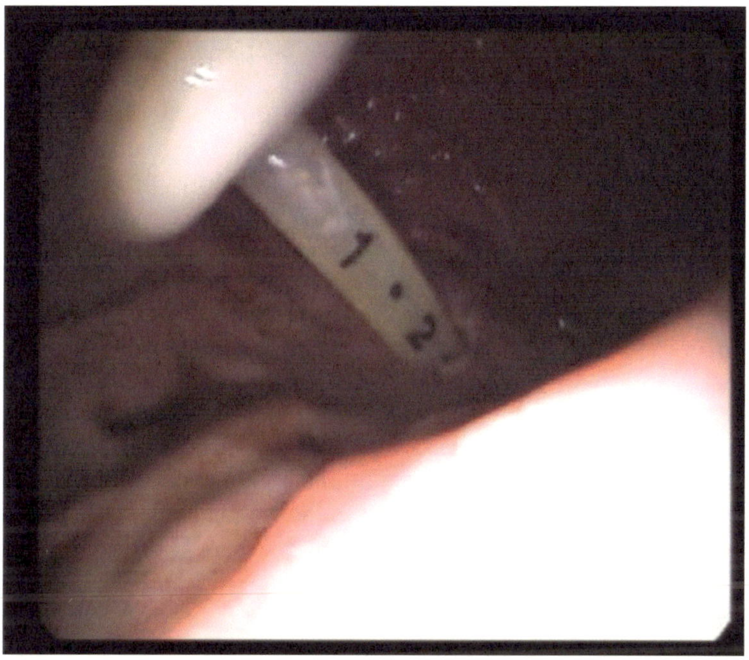

Fig. 3. PEG tube properly positioned, internal stomach view

3.2 Post-pyloric access

One concern about the use of nasogastric feeding in critically ill patients is the risk of reflux and aspiration of gastric contents; gastric reflux is often caused, however, by factors other than feeding (O'Keefe, 2009). These include sepsis, trauma, drugs, body position, gastroparesis, esophageal dysmotility, and obesity (O'Keefe, 2009). Gastric reflux, therefore, need not be a contraindication to gastric feeding; if gastric reflux persists despite the employment of preventative strategies, postpyloric enteral feeding may be employed (O'Keefe, 2009). Thus, in cases of gastroduodenal motility problems, pyloric stenosis or aspiration, a jejunal catheter, such as a PEG with jejunal extension (PEG/J) or direct percutaneous endoscopic jejunostomy (DPEJ), can be used (Niv et al., 2009; Kwon et al., 2010; Ho, 1983); such access systems can also be used to administer medications intra-jejunally, for example in therapy-resistant Parkinson's disease (Mathus-Vliegen, 2000). There are conflicting data in the recent literature about whether or not jejunal feeding definitely reduces the rate of reflux and aspiration (Loser et al., 2005; Finucane & Bynum, 1996; Lazarus et al., 1990; Mathus-Vliegen & Koning, 1999). Although PEJ was originally introduced to prevent aspiration, there remains a 2.4% risk of aspiration with post-pyloric feeding; the major indication for PEJ is significant impairment of gastric emptying (Cecil et al., 2008; Gutierrez & Balfe, 1991). No significant difference in inpatient mortality and length of stay was found in a recent observational study comparing PEG and PEJ (Poteet et al., 2010). PEJ insertion is also considered technically more demanding than PEG (Pearce et al., 2000). As an alternative to endoscopically-placed jejunostomy tubes, fluoroscopically-guided catheters can be placed. Percutaneous radiologic gastrojejunostomy (PRGJ) involves a longer and narrower tube than that placed in the stomach, and is thought to carry the potential for more frequent complications, such as tube blockage; PRGJ can be considered as a conversion from gastrostomy or placed as a primary option (Given et al., 2005; Shin & Park, 2010; Hoffer et al., 1999). Percutaneous radiologic jejunostomy (PRJ) is indicated in patients whose stomach is inaccessible for gastrostomy placement, or in those who have had a previous gastrectomy (Given et al., 2005; Shin & Park, 2010).

3.3 Surgical gastrostomy

Surgical gastrostomy is indicated for patients in whom PEG, RIG or PIG cannot be performed, or as an adjunctive procedure at the time the patient is undergoing surgery. Indications include esophageal atresia, stricture development, cancer, dysphagia due to neuromuscular disorders, or after trauma. Complications include local irritation, hemorrhage, skin excoriation from leaking of gastric contents, and wound infection. This procedure has largely been replaced by the PEG for its improved simplicity, and reduced costs (Pearce & Duncan, 2002). Surgical gastrostomy is technically simple but does involve an abdominal incision under general anesthesia. As most patients receiving surgical gastrostomy are malnourished, often with multiple medical problems, the operative risk is high and the gastrostomy site may heal poorly, causing leakage and not an insignificant amount of morbidity (Shellito & Malt, 1985).

4. Conclusion

Patients with neurologic dysfunction are at risk for malnourishment. The provision of supplemental nutrition, such as that afforded by percutaneous endoscopic gastrostomy, is potentially beneficial in many of these patients, but is not a risk-free procedure. Risks and benefits, ethical considerations, as well as the specific approach to be employed in any particular patient, must be weighed and discussed as part of the decision-making process. An awareness of the potential complications and their manifestations will both aid the clinician in advising patients about the decision to pursue gastrostomy, and help ensure a safer post-procedure course.

5. Acknowledgment

We would like to thank Dr. Joshua Vova, MD for his assistance with references in pediatric patients. We are also grateful to Mia White, reference librarian at Emory University, for her assistance with source formatting.

6. References

Al-Homaidhi, H.S.; & Tolia, V. (2001). Transverse colon volvulus around the gastrostomy tube site. *Journal of Pediatric Gastroenterology and Nutrition*, Vol. 33, No. 5, pp. 623-5

Alawadhi, A., Chou, S. & Soucy, P. (1991). Gastric volvulus--a late complication of gastrostomy. *Canadian Journal of Surgery*, Vol. 34, No. 5, pp. 485-6

Amann, W., Mischinger, H.J., Berger, A., Rosanelli, G., et al. (1997). Percutaneous endoscopic gastrostomy (PEG). 8 years of clinical experience in 232 patients. *Surgical Endoscopy*, Vol. 11, No. 7, pp. 741-4

American Society for Parenteral and Enteral Nutrition. (2002). Guidelines for the use of parenteral and enteral nutrition in adult and pediatric patients. *JPEN. Journal of Parenteral and Enteral Nutrition*, Vol. 26, No. 1 Suppl, pp. 1SA-138SA

Andersen, P.M., Borasio, G.D., Dengler, R., Hardiman, O., et al. (2007). Good practice in the management of amyotrophic lateral sclerosis: clinical guidelines. An evidence-based review with good practice points. EALSC Working Group. *Amyotrophic Lateral Sclerosis : Official publication of the World Federation of Neurology Research Group on Motor Neuron Diseases*, Vol. 8, No. 4, pp. 195-213

Annoni, J.M., Vuagnat, H., Frischknecht, R. & Uebelhart, D. (1998). Percutaneous endoscopic gastrostomy in neurological rehabilitation: a report of six cases. *Disability and Rehabilitation*, Vol. 20, No. 8, pp. 308-14

Barer, D.H. (1989). The natural history and functional consequences of dysphagia after hemispheric stroke. *Journal of Neurology, Neurosurgery, and Psychiatry*, Vol. 52, No. 2, pp. 236-41

Buchholz, D.W. (1994). Neurogenic dysphagia: what is the cause when the cause is not obvious? *Dysphagia*, Vol. 9, No. 4, pp. 245-55

Burke, D.T.; & Carayannopoulos, A.G. (2005). Percutaneous Endoscopic Gastrostomy Tube Placement Through the Transverse Colon of Stomach Causing Intractable Diarrhea: A Case Report. *American Journal of Physical Medicine and Rehabilitation*, Vol. 84, No. 3, pp. 222

Burke, D.T.; & Hoaglin, H. (2007). PEG Misplacement [Abstract]. *American Journal of Physical Medicine & Rehabilitation*, Vol. 86, No. 4, pp. S109

Burke, D.T.; & Geller, A.I. (2009). Peritonitis secondary to the migration of a trans-hepatically-placed percutaneous endoscopic gastrostomy tube: a case report. *Archives of Physical Medicine and Rehabilitation*, Vol. 90, No. 2, pp. 354-7

Burke, D.T., Hoberman, C.J., Morse, L.R. & Pina, B.D. (2005). A new procedure for gastrostomy tube replacement verification: a case report. *Archives of Physical Medicine and Rehabilitation*, Vol. 86, No. 7, pp. 1484-6

Burke, D.T., El Shami, A., Heinle, E. & Pina, B.D. (2006). Comparison of gastrostomy tube replacement verification using air insufflation versus gastrograffin. *Archives of Physical Medicine and Rehabilitation*, Vol. 87, No. 11, pp. 1530-3

Cappell, M.S.; & Abdullah, M. (2000). Management of gastrointestinal bleeding induced by gastrointestinal endoscopy. *Gastroenterology Clinics of North America*, Vol. 29, No. 1, pp. 125-67, vi-vii

Cecil, R.L., Goldman, L. & Ausiello, D.A. (2008). *Cecil medicine.* (23rd ed), Saunders Elsevier, 1416028056, Philadelphia

Cervo, F.A., Bryan, L. & Farber, S. (2006). To PEG or not to PEG: a review of evidence for placing feeding tubes in advanced dementia and the decision-making process. *Geriatrics*, Vol. 61, No. 6, pp. 30-5

Chernoff, R. (2006). Tube feeding patients with dementia. *Nutrition in Clinical Practice : official publication of the American Society for Parenteral and Enteral Nutrition*, Vol. 21, No. 2, pp. 142-6

Chio, A., Finocchiaro, E., Meineri, P., Bottacchi, E., et al. (1999). Safety and factors related to survival after percutaneous endoscopic gastrostomy in ALS. ALS Percutaneous Endoscopic Gastrostomy Study Group. *Neurology*, Vol. 53, No. 5, pp. 1123-5

Ciocon, J.O., Silverstone, F.A., Graver, L.M. & Foley, C.J. (1988). Tube feedings in elderly patients. Indications, benefits, and complications. *Archives of Internal Medicine*, Vol. 148, No. 2, pp. 429-33

de Baere, T., Chapot, R., Kuoch, V., Chevallier, P., et al. (1999). Percutaneous gastrostomy with fluoroscopic guidance: single-center experience in 500 consecutive cancer patients. *Radiology*, Vol. 210, No. 3, pp. 651-4

Deane, K.H., Whurr, R., Clarke, C.E., Playford, E.D., et al. (2001). Non-pharmacological therapies for dysphagia in Parkinson's disease. *Cochrane database of systematic reviews*, Vol. No. 1, pp. CD002816

Delegge, M.H. (2008). Percutaneous endoscopic gastrostomy in the dementia patient: helpful or hindering? *The American journal of gastroenterology*, Vol. 103, No. 4, pp. 1018-20

———. (2009). Tube feeding in patients with dementia: where are we? *Nutrition in Clinical Practice*, Vol. 24, No. 2, pp. 214-6

DeLegge, M.H., McClave, S.A., DiSario, J.A., Baskin, W.N., et al. (2005). Ethical and medicolegal aspects of PEG-tube placement and provision of artificial nutritional therapy. *Gastrointestinal Endoscopy*, Vol. 62, No. 6, pp. 952-9

Desport, J.C., Preux, P.M., Truong, T.C., Vallat, J.M., et al. (1999). Nutritional status is a prognostic factor for survival in ALS patients. *Neurology*, Vol. 53, No. 5, pp. 1059-63

Duszak, R., Jr.; & Mabry, M.R. (2003). National trends in gastrointestinal access procedures: an analysis of Medicare services provided by radiologists and other specialists. *Journal of Vascular and Interventional Radiology : JVIR*, Vol. 14, No. 8, pp. 1031-6

El-Matary, W. (2008). Percutaneous endoscopic gastrostomy in children. *Canadian Journal of Gastroenterology*, Vol. 22, No. 12, pp. 993-8

Finucane, T.E.; & Bynum, J.P. (1996). Use of tube feeding to prevent aspiration pneumonia. *Lancet*, Vol. 348, No. 9039, pp. 1421-4

Freeman, C., Ricevuto, A. & DeLegge, M.H. (2010). Enteral nutrition in patients with dementia and stroke. *Current Opinion in Gastroenterology*, Vol. 26, No. 2, pp. 156-9

Friedman, J.N., Ahmed, S., Connolly, B., Chait, P., et al. (2004). Complications associated with image-guided gastrostomy and gastrojejunostomy tubes in children. *Pediatrics*, Vol. 114, No. 2, pp. 458-61

Friedmann, R., Feldman, H. & Sonnenblick, M. (2007). Misplacement of percutaneously inserted gastrostomy tube into the colon: report of 6 cases and review of the literature. *JPEN. Journal of Parenteral and Enteral Nutrition*, Vol. 31, No. 6, pp. 469-76

Fröhlich, T., Richter, M., Carbon, R., Barth, B., et al. (2010). Review article: percutaneous endoscopic gastrostomy in infants and children. *Alimentary Pharmacology and Therapeutics*, Vol. 31, No. 8, pp. 788-801

Gaines, D.I., Durkalski, V., Patel, A. & DeLegge, M.H. (2009). Dementia and cognitive impairment are not associated with earlier mortality after percutaneous endoscopic gastrostomy. *JPEN. Journal of Parenteral and Enteral Nutrition*, Vol. 33, No. 1, pp. 62-6

Galaski, A., Peng, W.W., Ellis, M., Darling, P., et al. (2009). Gastrostomy tube placement by radiological versus endoscopic methods in an acute care setting: a retrospective review of frequency, indications, complications and outcomes. *Canadian Journal of Gastroenterology*, Vol. 23, No. 2, pp. 109-14

Galat, S.A., Gerig, K.D., Porter, J.A. & Slezak, F.A. (1990). Management of premature removal of the percutaneous gastrostomy. *The American Surgeon*, Vol. 56, No. 11, pp. 733-6

Garcia-Bueno, C.A., Rossi, T.M., Tjota, A., Camacho, C.A., et al. (1998). New insight on PEG tube placement in neurologically impaired patients. *Gastroenterology*, Vol. 114, No. Supplement 1, pp. A880-A880

Garrow, D., Pride, P., Moran, W., Zapka, J., et al. (2007). Feeding alternatives in patients with dementia: examining the evidence. *Clinical Gastroenterology and Hepatology : the official clinical practice journal of the American Gastroenterological Association*, Vol. 5, No. 12, pp. 1372-8

Gauderer, M.W., Ponsky, J.L. & Izant, R.J., Jr. (1980). Gastrostomy without laparotomy: a percutaneous endoscopic technique. *Journal of Pediatric Surgery*, Vol. 15, No. 6, pp. 872-5

Gencosmanoglu, R. (2004). Percutaneous endoscopic gastrostomy: a safe and effective bridge for enteral nutrition in neurological or non-neurological conditions. *Neurocritical Care*, Vol. 1, No. 3, pp. 309-17

Gillick, M.R. (2000). Rethinking the role of tube feeding in patients with advanced dementia. *The New England Journal of Medicine*, Vol. 342, No. 3, pp. 206-10

Given, M.F., Hanson, J.J. & Lee, M.J. (2005). Interventional radiology techniques for provision of enteral feeding. *Cardiovascular and Interventional Radiology*, Vol. 28, No. 6, pp. 692-703

Gomes, C.A., Jr., Lustosa, S.A., Matos, D., Andriolo, R.B., et al. (2010). Percutaneous endoscopic gastrostomy versus nasogastric tube feeding for adults with swallowing disturbances. *Cochrane database of systematic reviews*, Vol. No. 11, pp. CD008096

Gordon, C., Hewer, R.L. & Wade, D.T. (1987). Dysphagia in acute stroke. *British Medical Journal*, Vol. 295, No. 6595, pp. 411-4

Gossner, L., Keymling, J., Hahn, E.G. & Ell, C. (1999). Antibiotic prophylaxis in percutaneous endoscopic gastrostomy (PEG): a prospective randomized clinical trial. *Endoscopy*, Vol. 31, No. 2, pp. 119-24

Gramlich, L., Kichian, K., Pinilla, J., Rodych, N.J., et al. (2004). Does enteral nutrition compared to parenteral nutrition result in better outcomes in critically ill adult patients? A systematic review of the literature. *Nutrition*, Vol. 20, No. 10, pp. 843-8

Grant, M.D., Rudberg, M.A. & Brody, J.A. (1998). Gastrostomy placement and mortality among hospitalized Medicare beneficiaries. *JAMA : the journal of the American Medical Association*, Vol. 279, No. 24, pp. 1973-6

Green, C.J. (1999). Existence, causes and consequences of disease-related malnutrition in the hospital and the community, and clinical and financial benefits of nutritional intervention. *Clinical Nutrition*, Vol. 18, No. Supplement 2, pp. 3-28

Greff, M. (1999). Guidelines of the French Society of Digestive Endoscopy (SFED): endoscopic gastrostomy. *Endoscopy*, Vol. 31, No. 2, pp. 207-8

Gregory, S., Siderowf, A., Golaszewski, A.L. & McCluskey, L. (2002). Gastrostomy insertion in ALS patients with low vital capacity: respiratory support and survival. *Neurology*, Vol. 58, No. 3, pp. 485-7

Gutierrez, E.D.; & Balfe, D.M. (1991). Fluoroscopically guided nasoenteric feeding tube placement: results of a 1-year study. *Radiology*, Vol. 178, No. 3, pp. 759-62

Heyland, D.K., MacDonald, S., Keefe, L. & Drover, J.W. (1998). Total parenteral nutrition in the critically ill patient: a meta-analysis. *JAMA : the journal of the American Medical Association*, Vol. 280, No. 23, pp. 2013-9

Higaki, F., Yokota, O. & Ohishi, M. (2008). Factors predictive of survival after percutaneous endoscopic gastrostomy in the elderly: is dementia really a risk factor? *The American Journal of Gastroenterology*, Vol. 103, No. 4, pp. 1011-6; quiz 1017

Hill, K. (2008). Australian Clinical Guidelines for Acute Stroke Management 2007. *International journal of stroke : official journal of the International Stroke Society*, Vol. 3, No. 2, pp. 120-9

Ho, C.S. (1983). Percutaneous gastrostomy for jejunal feeding. *Radiology*, Vol. 149, No. 2, pp. 595-6

Hoffer, E.K., Cosgrove, J.M., Levin, D.Q., Herskowitz, M.M., et al. (1999). Radiologic gastrojejunostomy and percutaneous endoscopic gastrostomy: a prospective, randomized comparison. *Journal of Vascular and Interventional Radiology : JVIR*, Vol. 10, No. 4, pp. 413-20

Hogan, R.B., DeMarco, D.C., Hamilton, J.K., Walker, C.O., et al. (1986). Percutaneous endoscopic gastrostomy--to push or pull. A prospective randomized trial. *Gastrointestinal Endoscopy*, Vol. 32, No. 4, pp. 253-8

Horbach, T., Teske, V., Hohenberger, W. & Siassi, M. (2007). Endoscopic therapy of the buried bumper syndrome: a clinical algorithm. *Surgical Endoscopy*, Vol. 21, No. 8, pp. 1359-62

James, A., Kapur, K. & Hawthorne, A.B. (1998). Long-term outcome of percutaneous endoscopic gastrostomy feeding in patients with dysphagic stroke. *Age and Ageing*, Vol. 27, No. 6, pp. 671-6

James, R., Gines, D., Menlove, A., Horn, S.D., et al. (2005). Nutrition support (tube feeding) as a rehabilitation intervention. *Archives of Physical Medicine and Rehabilitation*, Vol. 86, No. 12 Suppl 2, pp. S82-S92

Katzberg, H.D.; & Benatar, M. (2011). Enteral tube feeding for amyotrophic lateral sclerosis/motor neuron disease. *Cochrane database of systematic reviews*, Vol. No. 1, pp. CD004030

Keohane, P.P., Atrill, H. & Silk, D.B. (1986). Clinical effectiveness of weighted and unweighted "fine-bore" nasogastric feeding tubes in enteral nutrition: a controlled clinical trial. *Journal of Clinical Nutrition and Gastroenterology*, Vol. No. 1, pp. 189–93

Khattak, I.U., Kimber, C., Kiely, E.M. & Spitz, L. (1998). Percutaneous endoscopic gastrostomy in paediatric practice: complications and outcome. *Journal of Pediatric Surgery*, Vol. 33, No. 1, pp. 67-72

Kidd, D., Lawson, J., Nesbitt, R. & MacMahon, J. (1995). The natural history and clinical consequences of aspiration in acute stroke. *QJM : monthly journal of the Association of Physicians*, Vol. 88, No. 6, pp. 409-13

Koretz, R.L., Avenell, A., Lipman, T.O., Braunschweig, C.L., et al. (2007). Does enteral nutrition affect clinical outcome? A systematic review of the randomized trials. *American Journal of Gastroenterology*, Vol. 102, No. 2, pp. 412-29; quiz 468

Kulick, D.; & Deen, D. (2011). Specialized nutrition support. *American Family Physician*, Vol. 83, No. 2, pp. 173-83

Kurien, M., McAlindon, M.E., Westaby, D. & Sanders, D.S. (2010). Percutaneous endoscopic gastrostomy (PEG) feeding. *BMJ*, Vol. 340, pp. c2414

Kwon, R.S., Banerjee, S., Desilets, D., Diehl, D.L., et al. (2010). Enteral nutrition access devices. *Gastrointestinal Endoscopy*, Vol. 72, No. 2, pp. 236-48

Laasch, H.U., Wilbraham, L., Bullen, K., Marriott, A., et al. (2003). Gastrostomy insertion: comparing the options--PEG, RIG or PIG? *Clinical Radiology*, Vol. 58, No. 5, pp. 398-405

Larson, D.E., Burton, D.D., Schroeder, K.W. & DiMagno, E.P. (1987). Percutaneous endoscopic gastrostomy. Indications, success, complications, and mortality in 314 consecutive patients. *Gastroenterology*, Vol. 93, No. 1, pp. 48-52

Lazarus, B.A., Murphy, J.B. & Culpepper, L. (1990). Aspiration associated with long-term gastric versus jejunal feeding: a critical analysis of the literature. *Archives of Physical Medicine and Rehabilitation*, Vol. 71, No. 1, pp. 46-53

Lee, J.H., Kim, J.J., Kim, Y.H., Jang, J.K., et al. (2002). Increased risk of peristomal wound infection after percutaneous endoscopic gastrostomy in patients with diabetes mellitus. *Digestive and Liver Disease : official journal of the Italian Society of Gastroenterology and the Italian Association for the Study of the Liver*, Vol. 34, No. 12, pp. 857-61

Lee, J.S., Jwa, C.S., Yi, H.J. & Chun, H.J. (2010). Impact of early enteral nutrition on in-hospital mortality in patients with hypertensive intracerebral hemorrhage. *Journal of Korean Neurosurgical Society*, Vol. 48, No. 2, pp. 99-104

Lee, L.; & MacPherson, M. (2010). Long-term percutaneous endoscopic gastrostomy feeding in young adults with multiple disabilities. *Internal Medicine Journal*, Vol. 40, No. 6, pp. 411-8

Leeds, J.S., McAlindon, M.E., Grant, J., Robson, H.E., et al. (2010). Survival analysis after gastrostomy: a single-centre, observational study comparing radiological and endoscopic insertion. *European Journal of Gastroenterology and Hepatology*, Vol. 22, No. 5, pp. 591-6

Lewis, C.L., Cox, C.E., Garrett, J.M., Hanson, L., et al. (2004). Trends in the use of feeding tubes in North Carolina hospitals. *Journal of General Internal Medicine*, Vol. 19, No. 10, pp. 1034-8

Lin, H.S., Ibrahim, H.Z., Kheng, J.W., Fee, W.E., et al. (2001). Percutaneous endoscopic gastrostomy: strategies for prevention and management of complications. *The Laryngoscope*, Vol. 111, No. 10, pp. 1847-52

Ljungdahl, M.; & Sundbom, M. (2006). Complication rate lower after percutaneous endoscopic gastrostomy than after surgical gastrostomy: a prospective, randomized trial. *Surgical Endoscopy*, Vol. 20, No. 8, pp. 1248-51

Loser, C., Aschl, G., Hebuterne, X., Mathus-Vliegen, E.M., et al. (2005). ESPEN guidelines on artificial enteral nutrition--percutaneous endoscopic gastrostomy (PEG). *Clinical Nutrition*, Vol. 24, No. 5, pp. 848-61

Luman, W., Kwek, K.R., Loi, K.L., Chiam, M.A., et al. (2001). Percutaneous endoscopic gastrostomy--indications and outcome of our experience at the Singapore General Hospital. *Singapore Medical Journal*, Vol. 42, No. 10, pp. 460-5

Maillet, J.O., Potter, R.L. & Heller, L. (2002). Position of the American Dietetic Association: ethical and legal issues in nutrition, hydration, and feeding. *Journal of the American Dietetic Association*, Vol. 102, No. 5, pp. 716-26

Marik, P.E.; & Zaloga, G.P. (2001). Early enteral nutrition in acutely ill patients: a systematic review. *Critical Care Medicine*, Vol. 29, No. 12, pp. 2264-70

Marshall, J.B., Bodnarchuk, G. & Barthel, J.S. (1994). Early accidental dislodgement of PEG tubes. *Journal of Clinical Gastroenterology*, Vol. 18, No. 3, pp. 210-2

Mathus-Vliegen, E.M. (2000). Gastrostomy and enterostomy, In: *Practice of Therapeutic Endoscopy*, Edited by G. N. J. Tytgat, M. Classen, J. D. Waye and S. Nakazawa. (2 ed), W.B. Saunders, 9780702025617, Philadelphia

Mathus-Vliegen, E.M., Koning, H., Taminiau, J.A. & Moorman-Voestermans, C.G. (2001). Percutaneous endoscopic gastrostomy and gastrojejunostomy in psychomotor retarded subjects: a follow-up covering 106 patient years. *Journal of Pediatric Gastroenterology and Nutrition*, Vol. 33, No. 4, pp. 488-94

Mathus-Vliegen, L.M.; & Koning, H. (1999). Percutaneous endoscopic gastrostomy and gastrojejunostomy: a critical reappraisal of patient selection, tube function and the feasibility of nutritional support during extended follow-up. *Gastrointestinal Endoscopy*, Vol. 50, No. 6, pp. 746-54

Mazzini, L., Corra, T., Zaccala, M., Mora, G., et al. (1995). Percutaneous endoscopic gastrostomy and enteral nutrition in amyotrophic lateral sclerosis. *Journal of Neurology*, Vol. 242, No. 10, pp. 695-8

McClave, S.A.; & Chang, W.K. (2003). Complications of enteral access. *Gastrointestinal Endoscopy*, Vol. 58, No. 5, pp. 739-51

McClave, S.A., Martindale, R.G., Vanek, V.W., McCarthy, M., et al. (2009). Guidelines for the Provision and Assessment of Nutrition Support Therapy in the Adult Critically Ill Patient: Society of Critical Care Medicine (SCCM) and American Society for Parenteral and Enteral Nutrition (A.S.P.E.N.). *JPEN. Journal of Parenteral and Enteral Nutrition*, Vol. 33, No. 3, pp. 277-316

McWhirter, J.P.; & Pennington, C.R. (1994). Incidence and recognition of malnutrition in hospital. *BMJ*, Vol. 308, No. 6934, pp. 945-8

Miller, R.E., Castlemain, B., Lacqua, F.J. & Kotler, D.P. (1989). Percutaneous endoscopic gastrostomy. Results in 316 patients and review of literature. *Surgical Endoscopy*, Vol. 3, No. 4, pp. 186-90

Mirtallo, J., Canada, T., Johnson, D., Kumpf, V., et al. (2004). Safe practices for parenteral nutrition. *JPEN. Journal of Parenteral and Enteral Nutrition*, Vol. 28, No. 6, pp. S39-70

Mitsumoto, H., Davidson, M., Moore, D., Gad, N., et al. (2003). Percutaneous endoscopic gastrostomy (PEG) in patients with ALS and bulbar dysfunction. *Amyotrophic Lateral Sclerosis Other Motor Neuron Disorders*, Vol. 4, No. 3, pp. 177-85

Mollitt, D.L., Dokler, M.L., Evans, J.S., Jeiven, S.D., et al. (1998). Complications of retained internal bolster after pediatric percutaneous endoscopic gastrostomy. *Journal of Pediatric Surgery*, Vol. 33, No. 2, pp. 271-3

Mularski, R.A., Sippel, J.M. & Osborne, M.L. (2000). Pneumoperitoneum: a review of nonsurgical causes. *Critical Care Medicine*, Vol. 28, No. 7, pp. 2638-44

Naik, R.P., Joshipura, V.P., Patel, N.R. & Haribhakti, S.P. (2009). Complications of PEG--prevention and management. *Tropical Gastroenterology : official journal of the Digestive Diseases Foundation*, Vol. 30, No. 4, pp. 186-94

National Collaborating Centre for Acute Care. (2006). In: *Nutrition Support for Adults: Oral Nutrition Support, Enteral Tube Feeding and Parenteral Nutrition*), National Collaborating Centre for Acute Care at The Royal College of Surgeons of England, 0954976029, London

Nicholson, F.B., Korman, M.G. & Richardson, M.A. (2000). Percutaneous endoscopic gastrostomy: a review of indications, complications and outcome. *Journal of Gastroenterology and Hepatology*, Vol. 15, No. 1, pp. 21-5

Nishiwaki, S., Araki, H., Shirakami, Y., Kawaguchi, J., et al. (2009). Inhibition of gastroesophageal reflux by semi-solid nutrients in patients with percutaneous endoscopic gastrostomy. *JPEN. Journal of Parenteral and Enteral Nutrition*, Vol. 33, No. 5, pp. 513-9

Niv, E., Fireman, Z. & Vaisman, N. (2009). Post-pyloric feeding. *World Journal of Gastroenterology : WJG*, Vol. 15, No. 11, pp. 1281-8

Niv, Y.; & Abuksis, G. (2003). Ethical aspects of percutaneous endoscopic gastrostomy insertion. *The Israel Medical Association journal : IMAJ*, Vol. 5, No. 3, pp. 212-3

Norman, K., Pichard, C., Lochs, H. & Pirlich, M. (2008). Prognostic impact of disease-related malnutrition. *Clinical Nutrition*, Vol. 27, No. 1, pp. 5-15

O'Keefe, S.J. (2009). A guide to enteral access procedures and enteral nutrition. *Nature Reviews. Gastroenterology & Hepatology*, Vol. 6, No. 4, pp. 207-15

O'Neill, P.A. (2000). Swallowing and prevention of complications. *British Medical Bulletin*, Vol. 56, No. 2, pp. 457-65

Orlando Regional Medical Center Department of Surgical Education. (October 2, 2009). Premature Gastrostomy / Jejunostomy Removal, Available from: <http://www.surgicalcriticalcare.net/Guidelines/premature%20gastrostomy%20removal%202009.pdf>

Ozmen, M.N.; & Akhan, O. (2002). Percutaneous radiologic gastrostomy. *European Journal of Radiology*, Vol. 43, No. 3, pp. 186-95

Palecek, E.J., Teno, J.M., Casarett, D.J., Hanson, L.C., et al. (2010). Comfort feeding only: a proposal to bring clarity to decision-making regarding difficulty with eating for persons with advanced dementia. *Journal of the American Geriatrics Society*, Vol. 58, No. 3, pp. 580-4

Park, J.H., Rhie, S. & Jeong, S.J. (2011). Percutaneous endoscopic gastrostomy in children. *Korean journal of Pediatrics*, Vol. 54, No. 1, pp. 17-21

Park, R.H., Allison, M.C., Lang, J., Spence, E., et al. (1992). Randomised comparison of percutaneous endoscopic gastrostomy and nasogastric tube feeding in patients with persisting neurological dysphagia. *BMJ*, Vol. 304, No. 6839, pp. 1406-9

Patwardhan, N., McHugh, K., Drake, D. & Spitz, L. (2004). Gastroenteric fistula complicating percutaneous endoscopic gastrostomy. *Journal of Pediatric Surgery*, Vol. 39, No. 4, pp. 561-4

Payne-James, J.; & Silk, D. (1988). Enteral nutrition: background, indications and management. *Bailliere's clinical gastroenterology*, Vol. 2, No. 4, pp. 815-47

Pearce, C.B.; & Duncan, H.D. (2002). Enteral feeding. Nasogastric, nasojejunal, percutaneous endoscopic gastrostomy, or jejunostomy: its indications and limitations. *Postgraduate Medical Journal*, Vol. 78, No. 918, pp. 198-204

Pearce, C.B., Goggin, P.M., Collett, J., Smith, L., et al. (2000). The 'cut and push' method of percutaneous endoscopic gastrostomy tube removal. *Clinical Nutrition*, Vol. 19, No. 2, pp. 133-5

Perel, P., Yanagawa, T., Bunn, F., Roberts, I., et al. (2006). Nutritional support for head-injured patients. *Cochrane database of systematic reviews*, Vol. No. 4, pp. CD001530

Phillips, N.M.; & Nay, R. (2008). A systematic review of nursing administration of medication via enteral tubes in adults. *Journal of Clinical Nursing*, Vol. 17, No. 17, pp. 2257-65

Potack, J.Z.; & Chokhavatia, S. (2008). Complications of and controversies associated with percutaneous endoscopic gastrostomy: report of a case and literature review. *Medscape Journal of Medicine*, Vol. 10, No. 6, pp. 142

Poteet, S.J., Holzman, M.D., Melvin, W.V., Sharp, K.W., et al. (2010). Inpatient mortality and length of stay comparison of percutaneous endoscopic gastrostomy and percutaneous endoscopic gastrojejunostomy. *Journal of Laparoendoscopic and Advanced Surgical Techniques. Part A*, Vol. 20, No. 7, pp. 587-90

Preshaw, R.M. (1981). A percutaneous method for inserting a feeding gastrostomy tube. *Surgery, Gynecology and Obstetrics*, Vol. 152, No. 5, pp. 658-60

Rabeneck, L., McCullough, L.B. & Wray, N.P. (1997). Ethically justified, clinically comprehensive guidelines for percutaneous endoscopic gastrostomy tube placement. *Lancet*, Vol. 349, No. 9050, pp. 496-8

Radunovic, A., Mitsumoto, H. & Leigh, P.N. (2007). Clinical care of patients with amyotrophic lateral sclerosis. *Lancet Neurology*, Vol. 6, No. 10, pp. 913-25

Rimon, E., Kagansky, N. & Levy, S. (2005). Percutaneous endoscopic gastrostomy; evidence of different prognosis in various patient subgroups. *Age and Ageing*, Vol. 34, No. 4, pp. 353-7

Ringleb, P.A., Bousser, M.G., Ford, G., Bath, P., et al. (2008). Guidelines for management of ischaemic stroke and transient ischaemic attack 2008. *Cerebrovascular Diseases*, Vol. 25, No. 5, pp. 457-507

Ritchie, C.S., Wilcox, C.M. & Kvale, E. (2007). Ethical and medicolegal issues related to percutaneous endoscopic gastrostomy placement. *Gastrointestinal Endoscopy Clinics of North America*, Vol. 17, No. 4, pp. 805-15

Roche, V. (2003). Percutaneous endoscopic gastrostomy. Clinical care of PEG tubes in older adults. *Geriatrics*, Vol. 58, No. 11, pp. 22-6, 28-9

Rosner, F. (1997). Guidelines for placement of percutaneous endoscopic gastrostomy tube. *Lancet*, Vol. 349, No. 9056, pp. 958

Safadi, B.Y., Marks, J.M. & Ponsky, J.L. (1998). Percutaneous endoscopic gastrostomy. *Gastrointestinal Endoscopy Clinics of North America*, Vol. 8, No. 3, pp. 551-68

Sampson, E.L., Candy, B. & Jones, L. (2009). Enteral tube feeding for older people with advanced dementia. *Cochrane database of systematic reviews*, Vol. No. 2, pp. CD007209

Schapiro, G.D.; & Edmundowicz, S.A. (1996). Complications of percutaneous endoscopic gastrostomy. *Gastrointestinal Endoscopy Clinics of North America*, Vol. 6, No. 2, pp. 409-22

Schrag, S.P., Sharma, R., Jaik, N.P., Seamon, M.J., et al. (2007). Complications related to percutaneous endoscopic gastrostomy (PEG) tubes. A comprehensive clinical review. *Journal of Gastrointestinal and Liver Diseases : JGLD*, Vol. 16, No. 4, pp. 407-18

Shellito, P.C.; & Malt, R.A. (1985). Tube gastrostomy. Techniques and complications. *Annals of Surgery*, Vol. 201, No. 2, pp. 180-5

Shin, J.H.; & Park, A.W. (2010). Updates on percutaneous radiologic gastrostomy/gastrojejunostomy and jejunostomy. *Gut and Liver*, Vol. 4 Suppl 1, No. pp. S25-31

Simpson, F.; & Doig, G.S. (2005). Parenteral vs. enteral nutrition in the critically ill patient: a meta-analysis of trials using the intention to treat principle. *Intensive Care Medicine*, Vol. 31, No. 1, pp. 12-23

Sleisenger, M.H., Feldman, M., Friedman, L.S. & Brandt, L.J. (2010). *Sleisenger and Fordtran's gastrointestinal and liver disease: pathophysiology, diagnosis, management*. Saunders/Elsevier, Retrieved from <http://www.mdconsult.com.proxy.library.emory.edu/books/page.do?eid=4-ul.0-B978-1-416>

Smithard, D.G., O'Neill, P.A., Parks, C. & Morris, J. (1996). Complications and outcome after acute stroke. Does dysphagia matter? *Stroke; a Journal of Cerebral Circulation*, Vol. 27, No. 7, pp. 1200-4

Spataro, R., Ficano, L., Piccoli, F. & La Bella, V. (2011). Percutaneous endoscopic gastrostomy in amyotrophic lateral sclerosis: Effect on survival. *Journal of the Neurological Sciences*, Vol. No. pp.

Srinivasan, R., Irvine, T. & Dalzell, M. (2009). Indications for percutaneous endoscopic gastrostomy and procedure-related outcome. *Journal of Pediatric Gastroenterology and Nutrition*, Vol. 49, No. 5, pp. 584-8

Srivastava, R., Stone, B.L. & Murphy, N.A. (2005). Hospitalist care of the medically complex child. *Pediatric Clinics of North America*, Vol. 52, No. 4, pp. 1165-87

Tao, H.H.; & Gillies, R.R. (1983). Percutaneous feeding gastrostomy. *AJR. American Journal of Roentgenology*, Vol. 141, No. 4, pp. 793-4

Vaisman, N., Lusaus, M., Nefussy, B., Niv, E., et al. (2009). Do patients with amyotrophic lateral sclerosis (ALS) have increased energy needs? *Journal of the Neurological Sciences*, Vol. 279, No. 1-2, pp. 26-9

Vervloessem, D., van Leersum, F., Boer, D., Hop, W.C., et al. (2009). Percutaneous endoscopic gastrostomy (PEG) in children is not a minor procedure: risk factors for major complications. *Seminars in Pediatric Surgery*, Vol. 18, No. 2, pp. 93-7

von Schnakenburg, C., Feneberg, R., Plank, C., Zimmering, M., et al. (2006). Percutaneous endoscopic gastrostomy in children on peritoneal dialysis. *Peritoneal Dialysis International : journal of the International Society for Peritoneal Dialysis*, Vol. 26, No. 1, pp. 69-77

Wicks, C., Gimson, A., Vlavianos, P., Lombard, M., et al. (1992). Assessment of the percutaneous endoscopic gastrostomy feeding tube as part of an integrated approach to enteral feeding. *Gut*, Vol. 33, No. 5, pp. 613-6

Wiesen, A.J., Sideridis, K., Fernandes, A., Hines, J., et al. (2006). True incidence and clinical significance of pneumoperitoneum after PEG placement: a prospective study. *Gastrointestinal Endoscopy*, Vol. 64, No. 6, pp. 886-9

Wills, J.S.; & Oglesby, J.T. (1983). Percutaneous gastrostomy. *Radiology*, Vol. 149, No. 2, pp. 449-53

Wilson, W.C., Zenone, E.A. & Spector, H. (1990). Small intestinal perforation following replacement of a percutaneous endoscopic gastrostomy tube. *Gastrointestinal Endoscopy*, Vol. 36, No. 1, pp. 62-3

Ziegler, T.R. (2009). Parenteral nutrition in the critically ill patient. *The New England Journal of Medicine*, Vol. 361, No. 11, pp. 1088-97

5

Defining the Indications for Prophylactic Percutaneous Endoscopic Gastrostomy Tubes in Surgically Treated Head and Neck Cancer Patients

Jason Foster[1], Peter Filocamo[1], William Brady[2],
Thom Loree[1] and John F. Gibbs[1]
*[1]Department of Surgery, Roswell Park Cancer Institute,
State University of New York at Buffalo, Elm & Carlton Streets, Buffalo, NY
[2]Department of Biostatics, Roswell Park Cancer Institute,
State University of New York at Buffalo, Elm & Carlton Streets, Buffalo, NY
U.S.A.*

1. Introduction

Malnutrition is a common problem in head and neck cancer with up to 50% of the patients developing some degree of nutritional deficiency.[1] The etiologies of this problem can be divided into two categories: tumor related or treatment related. Patient with tumor related malnutrition typically present with obvious clinical signs and symptoms of undernourishment. Tumor cachexia can contribute but this is primarily caused by physical impediments to oral consumption such as pain, oropharygeal obstruction, or nerve compression , all resulting in discordant degluttination.[2] Prior to definitive cancer therapy, this group of patients requires nutritional resuscitation.

Additionally many patients who present nutritionally sound and who undergo surgical resection experience some degree of postoperative nutritional difficulties. In many cases it a short lived and inconsequential. However, a subset of patients will experience a more severe prolonged course requiring enteral supplementation. Prior studies have shown that if these patients are not supplemented, they will likely experience severe dehydration, treatment intolerance, or severe treatment related complications that require hospitalization.[3,4] Inherently, the surgical treatment of head and neck malignancies can be quite debilitating and result in significant mastication and deglutination dysfunction.[5-7] At times this involves radical resections that require complex reconstructions to maintain oropharyngeal continuity; and adjuvant radiation and/or chemotherapy may be required to maximize local control. Indiscriminately placing PEG tubes in all patients would put many patients at risk for PEG related complications.[8-13] Therefore, the difficulty has been trying to preoperatively identify which patients likely to experience prolonged treatment induced malnutrition and benefit from early nutritional supplementation.

Groups have identified some factors that are predictive of a need for enteral support.[3,4,14-17] One factor that has been clearly established is radiation therapy, particular when given postoperatively.[3,4,17] Other factors such as Stage IV disease, base of tongue tumor location, and heavy alcohol ingestion are less clearly defined.[14-16] Some criticisms have been that the studies conducted to identify these variables were small, used a mixed population of surgical and non-surgical patients, and often used durations of enteral support that were short (< 4 weeks) or undefined.

At Roswell Park Cancer Institute (RPCI) prophylactic PEG are routinely placed in surgically treated patients who require a composite resection, flap reconstruction, radiation therapy, chemotherapy, and at the discretion of the attending surgical staff. We found that many patients required their PEG tube for 4 weeks or less; while some patients required their PEG for a year or longer. In order to more accurately define which patients benefited from prophylactic PEG placement we reviewed our experience. We used a homogenous population of surgically treated head and neck cancer patients to identified patient, tumor, and treatment factors that were predictive of a short-term (≤ 3 months) and long-term (≥1 year) PEG tube dependency.

2. Methods

One hundred forty one cases of surgically treated head and neck cancers treated at RPCI from January 1, 1999 to December 31, 2003 who underwent pretreatment placement of PEG tubes were reviewed. Only patients with squamous cell carcinoma (SCC) of the oral cavity, oropharynx, larynx, and pharynx were included in this study eliminating 14 patients. Seven patients had PEG tube placed a second time for the treatment of a new primary or recurrent disease, and six patients did not have complete records, leaving 114 patients for evaluation.

The variables analyzed were divided into patient factors (age and sex), tumor factors (primary site, T stage and nodal status), and treatment factors (flap reconstruction, radiation, and chemotherapy). A short-term dependency required that the PEG tube be in place for 3 months or less, while a long-term dependency require usage for a year or longer.

2.1 Statistical method

The duration of PEG tube dependency was calculated from the date of placement until the time of removal. Patients who had their PEG tube removed and not replaced were considered to be no longer dependent on it. Patients who died while still dependent on their PEG tube, or who were still dependent at last documented follow-up were considered to have censored durations. Because of this censoring, time to event analyses was used. The distribution of PEG duration was compared across age, sex, tumor sites, T stage, N stage, flap reconstruction, radiation, and chemotherapy. Kaplan-Meier estimates of the proportions (and 95% confidence intervals {CIs}) of patients with PEG tubes in place at 3 and 12 months after placement were determined for each variable and log-rank tests were used to compare durations.

Proportional hazards regression models were used to compare durations while accounting for other factors. Variables were selected for inclusion in the model in a stepwise selection process. Variables were entered in the model if $p<0.05$ and were retained if $p<0.05$. Because a number of patients had unknown T stage (8 patients) and unknown N stage (20 patients), in the proportional hazards regression models, these factors included separate levels for 'unknown' T and 'unknown' N stage, respectively. In the log-rank analyses of T stages and N stages, patients with unknown stages were not included.

These analyses are post hoc so no adjustments for multiplicity are made. All tests were done two-sided with a significance level of 0.05. All analyses were done using SAS version 8.2.

3. Results

The mean age of patients in this study was 65 and 65% of patients were male. Sixty-four percent of the patients had advanced T stage or recurrent disease and node positive disease was present in 49% of the patients. Flap reconstructions were performed in 39% of patients, while the rate of adjuvant therapy was 40% for radiation and 11% for chemotherapy. The percentage of patients in each of the four major tumor sites were 42% oral cavity, 23% oropharynx, 26% larynx, and 9% pharynx. In Table 1 the patient characteristics (age, sex), tumor characteristics (T stage, N stage), and treatment (flap reconstruction, radiation, chemotherapy) characteristic, along with PEG status at the end of the study is presented for each major tumor site. Overall 64% (73/114) of patients in the study had their PEG tubes removed.

Sixty-nine percent of patients had short-term PEG usage. When the group receiving adjuvant radiation was compared to the group that did not receive radiation treatment a significant difference was observed 91% (83, 99) vs. 53% (41, 65). Eighty-nine percent of pharyngeal tumor site patient and 92% of chemotherapy patients had a short term dependency but this was not statistically different from the other tumors site or the no chemotherapy group respectively. The short-term dependency was not influenced by patient age, sex, T stage, N stage, or flap reconstruction (Table 2).

The long-term dependency for this group of patients was 36%. Table 2 presents Kaplan-Meier estimates of the proportions of patients with PEG tubes in place at 12 months for each variable. PEG tube duration was statistically significantly different across surgical sites: 78% of pharynx patients still had their tubes in place after 12 months, while only 45% of oral cavity patients, 34% of oropharynx patients, and 11% or larynx patients had tubes in place. Patients who underwent flap reconstruction also had statistically significantly (p=0.004) longer PEG tube durations than those who did not, 52% vs. 25%, respectively. When a multivariate analysis was performed, adjusting for other factors, site and flap reconstruction remained as statistically significantly long-term risk factors. Chemotherapy was also found to be significant factor in long-term PEG dependency.

4. Discussion

The prevention of malnutrition and early nutritional support in the management of cancer patients is well documented. Specifically in head and neck cancer, suboptimal nutrition during definitive treatment results in a significant increase in surgical complications, dehydration, therapy breaks and hospitalizations. (3). Because malnutrition can result in reduced immunosurvelliance, it may contribute to early local and distant cancer recurrence. (18, 19) Avoidance of treatment induced malnutrition may prevent these complications, and prophylactic placement of PEG tube provides access for the delivery of nutrition. Identification of the risk factors which contribute to prolonged enteral support ensures PEG placement in the appropriate patients. Of equal importance is that accurate risk factors can avoids subjecting low risk patients to PEG related complications, and costs. In this study we found that radiation was the only predictor of a short-term dependency; while pharyngeal tumor site, flap reconstruction, and chemotherapy were predictive a long-term need.

	Site									
	Oral cavity		Oropharynx		Larynx		Pharynx			
	n	%	n	%	n	%	n	%	n	%
All	49		26		30		9		114	
Removal Category										
Died	10	20	5	19	2	7	6	67	23	20
In Use at End of Follow-up	11	22	4	15	1	3	1	11	17	15
Removed	28	57	17	65	26	87	2	22	73	64
Unknown/Loss to Follow-up	0	0	0	0	1	3	0	0	1	1
Age, PEG Placed (y)										
<55	10	20	9	35	7	23	2	22	28	25
55-64	10	20	8	31	12	40	3	33	33	29
65-74	16	33	6	23	7	23	3	33	32	28
>=75	13	27	3	12	4	13	1	11	21	18
Sex										
F	24	49	5	19	8	27	3	33	40	35
M	25	51	21	81	22	73	6	67	74	65
Chemotherapy										
Unknown	1	2	0	0	0	0	0	0	1	1
No	46	94	22	85	24	80	9	100	101	89
Yes	2	4	4	15	6	20	0	0	12	11
Radiation										
Unknown	1	2	0	0	0	0	0	0	1	1
No	32	65	11	42	19	63	5	56	67	59
Yes	16	33	15	58	11	37	4	44	46	40
Flap Reconstruction										
No	34	69	7	27	25	83	3	33	69	61
Yes	15	31	19	73	5	17	6	67	45	39
T Stage										
Unknown	3	6	3	12	2	7	0	0	8	7
Recurrence	14	29	7	27	9	30	0	0	30	26
T1	2	4	1	4	2	0	2	22	5	4
T2	16	33	6	23	5	17	1	11	28	25
T3	5	10	7	27	11	37	4	44	27	24
T4	9	18	2	8	3	10	2	22	16	14
Node Involvement										
Unknown	6	12	6	23	6	20	0	0	18	16
No	21	43	2	8	13	43	4	44	40	35
Yes	22	45	18	59	11	37	5	56	56	49

Table 1. Characteristics of Patients by Surgical Site

	N ¶	Median Duration (95% CI)	Percent† (95% CI) of Patients With PEG at		p (log-rank)	p for selected covariates ‡
			3 months	12 months		
Site						
Oral cavity	49	11.2 (4.1, NE)	64% (51%, 78%)	45% (31%, 60%)	0.007	0.004
Oropharynx	26	6.6 (4.0, 18.2)	80% (64%, 96%)	34% (15%, 53%)		
Larynx	30	3.5 (2.6, 5.9)	62% (45%, 80%)	11% (0%, 23%)		
Pharynx	9	NE	89% (68%, 100%)	78% (51%, 100%)		
Age, PEG Placed (y)						
<55	28	7.1 (4.7, 11.3)	78% (63%, 94%)	29% (11%, 47%)	0.157	NA
55-64	33	3.1 (2.3, 6.6)	52% (34%, 69%)	26% (10%, 41%)		
65-74	32	11.2 (5.0, NE)	87% (75%, 99%)	50% (31%, 68%)		
≥75	21	4.4 (2.6, 19.1)	60% (38%, 81%)	41% (18%, 64%)		
Sex						
F	40	5.0 (4.0, 11.2)	68% (54%, 83%)	32% (16%, 48%)	0.583	NA
M	74	6.6 (4.9, 11.3)	70% (59%, 80%)	37% (25%, 49%)		
Radiation						
No	67	3.2 (2.3, 8.7)	53% (41%, 65%)	34% (22%, 46%)	0.102	NA
Yes	46	8.2 (6.6, 13.8)	91% (83%, 99%)	38% (23%, 53%)		
Chemotherapy						
No	101	5.9 (4.1, 8.7)	66% (57%, 76%)	35% (25%, 44%)	0.141	<0.001
Yes	12	10.6 (4.9, NE)	92% (76%, 100%)	46% (17%, 76%)		
Flap Reconstruction						
No	69	4.9 (2.7, 6.6)	62% (50%, 73%)	24% (13%, 35%)	0.002	0.011
Yes	45	18.2 (5.6, NE)	82% (70%, 93%)	54% (38%, 69%)		
T Stage						
Recurrence	30	5.9 (2.7, 18.2)	66% (49%, 83%)	42% (22%, 61%)	0.151	NA
T1	5	NE	80% (45%, 100%)	53% (5%, 100%)		
T2	28	6.3 (3.8, 11.3)	71% (55%, 88%)	27% (9%, 45%)		
T3	27	5.0 (2.6, 9.9)	66% (48%, 84%)	24% (7%, 41%)		
T4	16	NE	80% (60%, 100%)	60% (35%, 85%)		
Node Involvement						
No	40	5.4 (2.6, 8.7)	62% (47%, 77%)	33% (18%, 49%)	0.663	NA
Yes	56	6.6 (4.7, 11.2)	74% (63%, 86%)	30% (18%, 43%)		

¶ At PEG placement.
† Percents and medians are Kaplan-Meier estimates.
‡ From likelihood ratio tests for selected covariates from proportional hazards regression models using stepwise selection.
NA = not applicable (term not selected for inclusion in proportional hazards regression model).
NE = not estimable

Table 2. Time-to-Event Analyses of PEG Duration

Other groups have documented that radiation treatment results in significant malnutrition.(3,4,20) Radiation treatment often results in xerostomia, loss of taste, mucositis, and tumor edema which all contribute to poor oral intake and nutritional deficits. When patients receive primary radiation without nutritional support 40% of patient loose more than 10% of their baseline weights, 40% of patients require hospitalization during the treatment with 20% of patients requiring therapy break, and 40% of these patients will require a gastrostomy placement to complete therapy. (3,4,20) As expected 91% of patients who received radiation in addition to surgical resection required short term enteral support. However, this dependency was self-limited, and did not impact long term oral nutrition, evident by no difference at 1 year between the radiated or unirradiated (Table 2).

A pharyngeal site was significant on univariate analysis, while flap reconstruction was significant on both univariate and multivariate analysis. Given the significant amount of dysfunction associated with these surgical procedures, this data validates our clinical expectation that these subsets benefit from prophylactic PEGs. Importantly, given the propensity of oral pharyngeal bacterial overgrowth in this patient subset and significant intra-oral tumor burden, we believe that the T-fastener technique should be used to prevent/reduce PEG site abscess and local cancer recurrence. We previously published that the T-fastener technique has a low rate of local infection and cancer recurrence in head and neck carcinoma population. (21)

Chemotherapy was the only other significant factor on multivariate analysis. Although our series was small, the increasing use of chemotherapy in the management of the head and neck SCC population will dramatically increase this patient fraction requiring nutritional support. In our study almost half of chemotherapy patients required long-term support. We believe that prophylactic PEG placement should be part of the management discussion in patients receiving adjuvant or neoadjuvant chemotherapy.

Importantly when PEG tubes are placed in this patient population, the usage of the T-fastener technique is critical. Most of these patients are at high risk for PEG site infection and tumor implantation when the pull through technique is used in this patient population. We recently published that the rate of these complications can be significantly reduced by direct PEG placement with T-fastener strategy.

This review confirmed the favorable current approach to prophylactic PEG tube in the head and neck cancer population. Aside from patients who present malnourished, prophylactic PEG tubes should be placed in all SCC head and neck cancer patients who have a pharyngeal primary tumor site, require flap reconstruction, undergo radiation therapy, and/or chemotherapy.

5. References

[1] Bassett MR, Dobie RA: Patterns of nutritional deficiency in head and neck cancer. *Otolaryngol Head Neck Surg* 91:119-25, 1983

[2] Logemann JA, Bytell DE: Swallowing disorders in three types of head and neck surgical patients. *Cancer* 44:1095-105, 1979

[3] Fietkau R, Iro H, Sailer D, et al: Percutaneous endoscopically guided gastrostomy in patients with head and neck cancer. *Recent Results Cancer Re*s 121:269-82, 1991

[4] Lee JH, Machtay M, Unger LD, et al: Prophylactic gastrostomy tubes in patients undergoing intensive irradiation for cancer of the head and neck. *Arch Otolaryngol Head Neck Surg* 124:871-5, 1998

[5] Martini DV, Har-El G, Lucente FE, et al: Swallowing and pharyngeal function in postoperative pharyngeal cancer patients. *Ear Nose Throat J* 76:450-3, 456, 1997

[6] Vokes EE, Kies MS, Haraf DJ, et al: Concomitant chemoradiotherapy as primary therapy for locoregionally advanced head and neck cancer. *J Clin Oncol* 18:1652-61, 2000

[7] Murry T, Madasu R, Martin A, et al: Acute and chronic changes in swallowing and quality of life following intraarterial chemoradiation for organ preservation in patients with advanced head and neck cancer. *Head Neck* 20:31-7, 1998

[8] Baredes S, Behin D, Deitch E: Percutaneous endoscopic gastrostomy tube feeding in patients with head and neck cancer. *Ear Nose Throat* J 83:417-9, 2004

[9] Ehrsson YT, Langius-Eklof A, Bark T, et al: Percutaneous endoscopic gastrostomy (PEG) - a long-term follow-up study in head and neck cancer patients. *Clin Otolaryngol Allied Sci* 29:740-6, 2004

[10] Hunter JG: Tumor implantation at PEG exit sites in head and neck cancer patients: how much evidence is enough? *J Clin Gastroenterol* 37:280, 2003

[11] Sharma P, Berry SM, Wilson K, et al: Metastatic implantation of an oral squamous-cell carcinoma at a percutaneous endoscopic gastrostomy site. *Surg Endosc* 8:1232-5, 1994

[12] van Erpecum KJ, Akkersdijk WL, Warlam-Rodenhuis CC, et al: Metastasis of hypopharyngeal carcinoma into the gastrostomy tract after placement of a percutaneous endoscopic gastrostomy catheter. *Endoscopy* 27:124-7, 1995

[13] Tucker AT, Gourin CG, Ghegan MD, et al: 'Push' versus 'pull' percutaneous endoscopic gastrostomy tube placement in patients with advanced head and neck cancer. *Laryngoscope* 113:1898-902, 2003

[14] Gardine RL, Kokal WA, Beatty JD, et al: Predicting the need for prolonged enteral supplementation in the patient with head and neck cancer. *Am J Surg* 156:63-5, 1988

[15] Anwander T, Berge S, Appel T, et al: Percutaneous endoscopic gastrostomy for long-term feeding of patients with oropharyngeal tumors. *Nutr Cancer* 50:40-5, 2004

[16] Schweinfurth JM, Boger GN, Feustel PJ: Preoperative risk assessment for gastrostomy tube placement in head and neck cancer patients. *Head Neck* 23:376-82, 2001

[17] Scolapio JS, Spangler PR, Romano MM, et al: Prophylactic placement of gastrostomy feeding tubes before radiotherapy in patients with head and neck cancer: is it worthwhile? *J Clin Gastroenterol* 33:215-7, 2001

[18] van Bokhoust-de van der Schuer, von Blomberg-van der Flier BM, Kuik DJ, Klop, Scholten PE, Siroen MP, Snow GB, Quak, JJ, van Leeuwen PA . Survival of malnourished head and neck cancer patients can be predicted by human leukocyte antigen-DR expression and interleukin-6/tumor necreosis factor-alpha response of the monocyte. *J Parenter Enteral Nutr.* 24(6):, 329-36, 2000

[19] van Bokhoust-de van der Schuer, van Leeuwen PA, Kuik DJ, Klop WM, Sauerwein HP, Snow GB, Quak, JJ. The impact of nutritional status on the prognoses of patients with advanced head and neck cancer. *Cancer* 86(3): 519-27, 1999

[20] Jensen K, Lambertsen K, Grau C. Late swallowing dysfunction and dysphagia after radiotherapy for pharynx cancer: frequency, intensity and correlation with dose and volume parameters. *Radiother Oncol* 85(1): 74-82, 2007.

[21] Foster J, Filacoma P, Brady W, Nava H, Hicks W, Loree T, Rigual N, Smith J, Gibbs JF. The introducer technique is a safe method for placing percutaneous endoscopic gastrostomy tubes in head and neck cancer patients. *Surg Endos* 21: 897-01, 2006

Part 3

Gastrostomy Techniques

6

The Place of Laparoscopic Gastrostomy in the Surgical Armamentarium

Philip Ng Cheng Hin
Department Of Surgery, University Hospital Lewisham, London
UK

1. Introduction

Historically, gastrostomy has been performed for centuries and recently with the advent of Laparoscopic surgery, laparoscopic gastrostomy (ref 1) has been added to the options available to surgeons.

Laparoscopic gastrostomy can be considered when other minimally invasive methods such as PEG (Percutaneous Endoscopic Gastrostomy) is not feasible or fails. PEG can be come impossible if the endoscope cannot be introduced, because of physical or functional obstruction. The alternative is to consider PRG (Percutaneous Radiologically Guided) insertion prior to considering open gastrostomy via laparotomy, (LG) Laparoscopic gastrostomy has carved itself an important niche in that respect.

2. Indications of gastrostomy

a. Patients requiring Medium or long term feeding
- Starvation
- Swallowing problems, long term neurological conditions
- Chronic problems in children e.g. mucoviscidosis, reflux
- Impassable benign or malignant stricture

b. Decompression of the stomach
c. Gastric access
d. Failure of PEG
e. Failure of PRG

3. Contra indications

a. Unfit patients who cannot lie flat.
b. Abdominal access not possible due to previous operations or gross obesity, fixed flexion deformity.

4. Techniques

a. Double puncture laparoscopic assisted gastrostomy (ref 2, 4)

Once the abdomen prepped, entry into the peritoneal cavity is performed using any preferred technique through a periumbilical port and the pneumoperitoneum is established, the anterior wall of the stomach is identified with certainty, and a second port (10mm) is inserted at a convenient point on the anterior abdominal wall. This operative step is greatly assisted by changing the position of the operating table 20 degrees head up. Once the anterior gastric wall is identified, it is firmly grasped using a Babcock forceps and withdrawn slowly through the port site while the abdomen is deflated. (Fig1)

The stomach usually comes easily to be exteriorised through the port site, which is then enlarged.

Two concentric purse strings of 2/0 PDS are inserted on the gastric wall, (fig 2) keeping the needles attached and a small gastrotomy performed using either diathermy or a No 11 blade. (Fig3)

The appropriate size gastrostomy tube or button can then be inserted (Fig 4) and the retaining balloon inflated. The two purse strings are tied securely, creating a small well, and the needles used to attach the stomach wall to the anterior abdominal. Two extra stitches are then used to secure the stomach wall to the anterior abdominal wall as in a 4-point fixation. The correct intragastric position of the feeding tube is then verified by reinflating the peritoneal cavity slowly to 5mm Hg. (Fig 5) The patency and absence of leakage is then tested with the laparoscope in situ and if satisfactory, the entry port is closed after deflation. Feeding can start immediately at 30-ml/ hour increasing to 60ml/hr, then full feed. Local anaesthetic is infiltrated into the wounds as required.

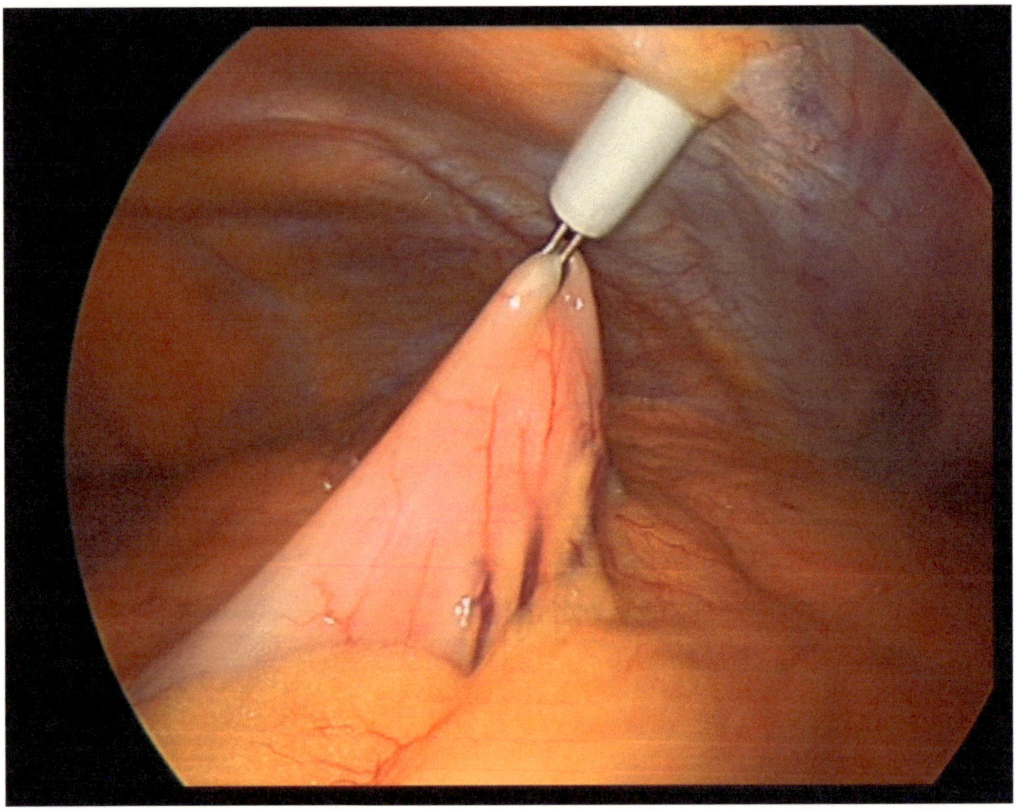

Fig. 1.

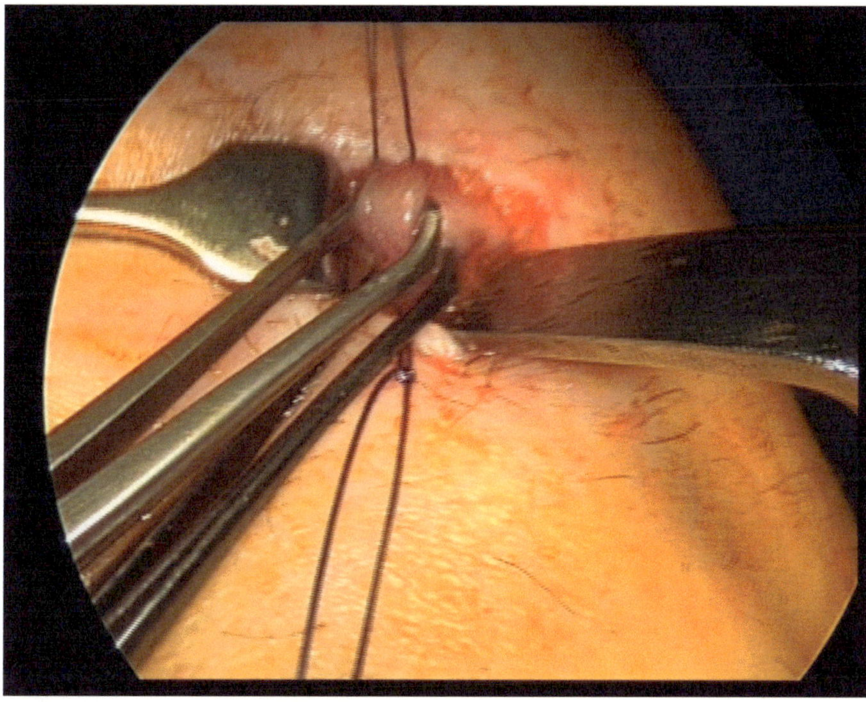

Fig. 2.

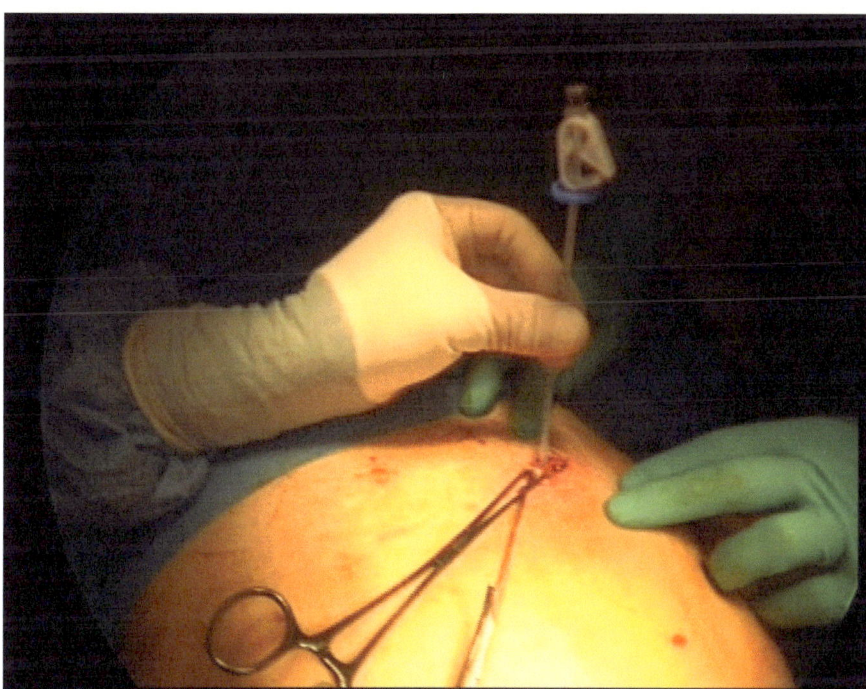

Fig. 3.

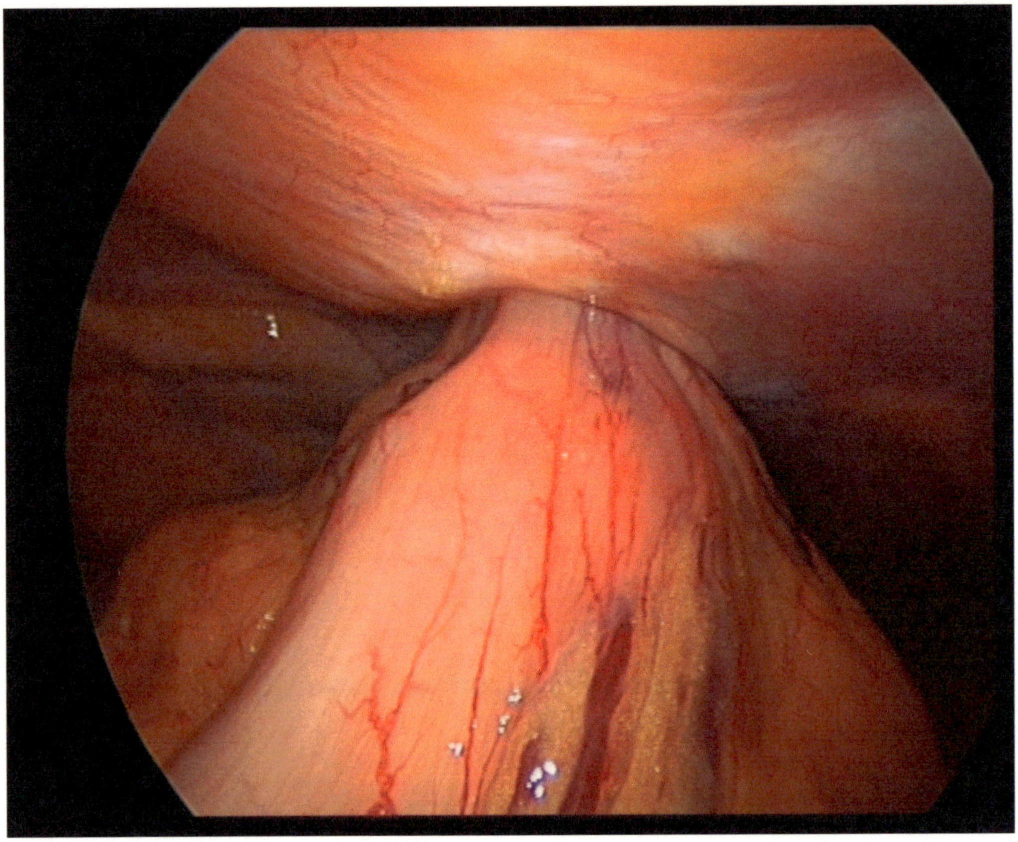

Fig. 4.

b. Single puncture laparoscopic assisted gastrostomy

In the Single puncture technique, the site of the gastrostomy is chosen first. Either local anaesthetic is infiltrated or a general anaesthetic administered to allow access to the abdominal cavity is achieved. A 10 mm trocar is used to carry a 10 mm scope and an operating laparoscope with an instrument channel is used. After identification of the anterior gastric wall, a forceps is used to grasp the anterior gastric wall, which is then exteriorised as the abdomen is deflated. The gastrotomy can be performed between two concentric purse strings as in the double puncture technique, its position inside the stomach ascertained and the tube secured in the same manner.

c. Button laparoscopic gastrostomy

The technique here is also similar to the gastrostomy technique substituting the button for the gastrostomy tube (Ref 5). A useful measure is to first insert a Foley catheter into the gastrotomy and mark the level (Fig5) in order to measure the exact size of button.

Once the button gastrostomy tube has been inserted, the purse strings tied, and the balloon inflated, the correct intragastric position can be verified by reinflating the abdomen to a pressure of 5mm Hg and tugging on the tube while checking the position under direct vision.(fig6)

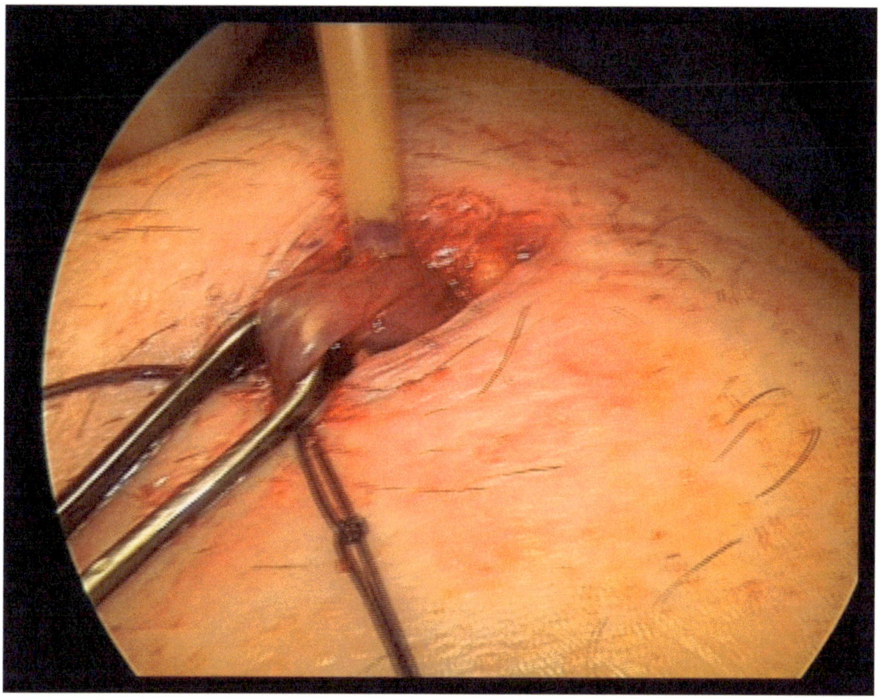

Fig. 5.

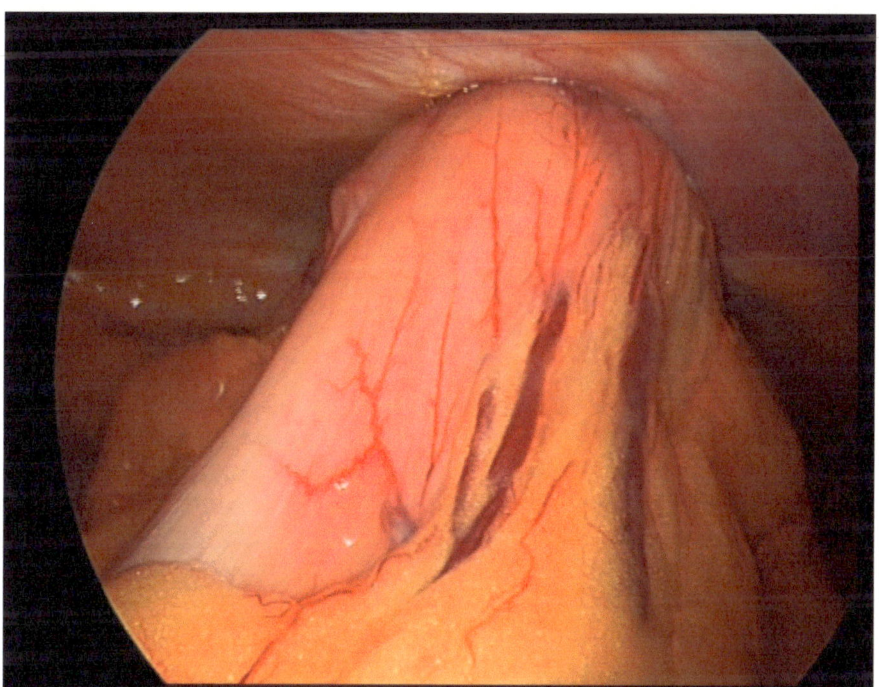

Fig. 6.

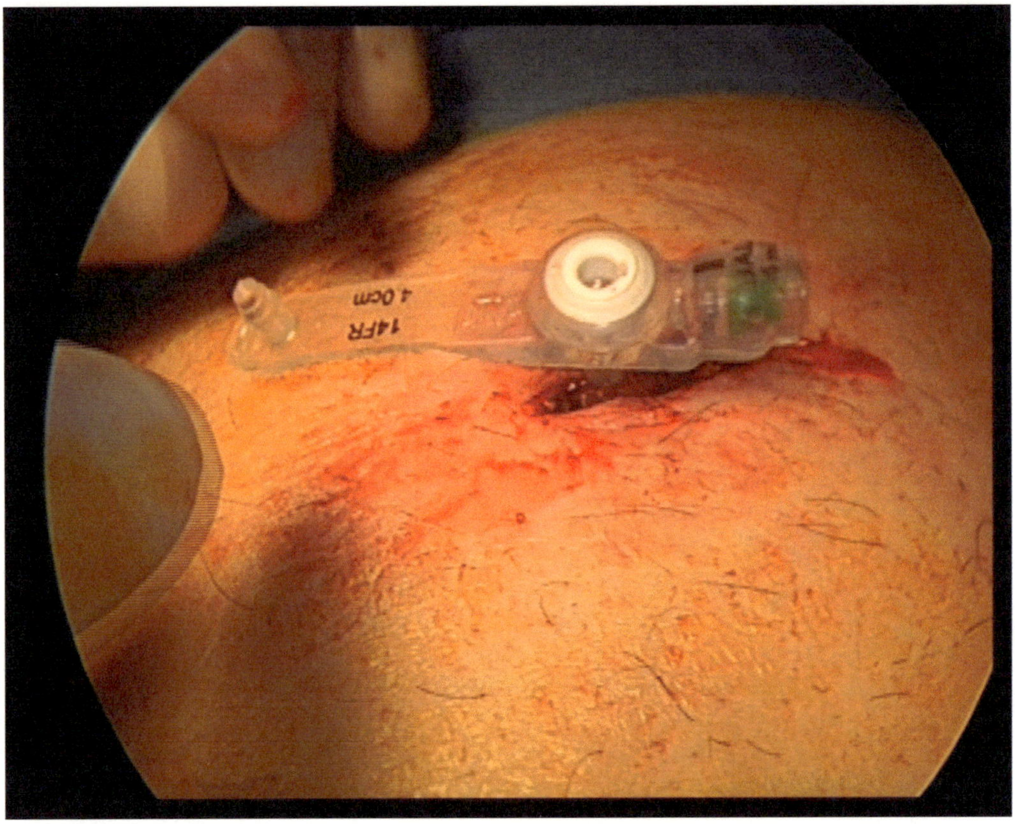

Fig. 7.

5. Anaesthetic

Local infiltration, Loco regional or general can be used

a. General anaesthetic with or without muscle relaxant although use of the latter facilitates rapid exploration and identification of intra abdominal organs.
b. Loco regional
c. Spinal anaesthetic where indicated
d. Local and sedation
e. Where neither General nor loco regional is indicated simple local anaesthetic can be used with success after careful infiltration of anaesthetic such as Xylocaine 1% in the tissues prior to cutting. Sedation is useful to keep the patient compliant. A preset pressure of 5-10mm Hg is adequate for laparoscopic visualisation.
f. Local only. When all other options cannot be used just simple infiltration can be used in thin patients.

6. Patient position

The ideal patient position is flat on the operating table with a 20 degree head up tilt. Patients who have problems straightening their spine may prove difficult to access. Patients with fixed flexion deformity of the hip may prove difficult to scope, in which case, a 20 degree left side up tilt table rotation may prove useful.

7. Consent

The 30-day mortality in most studies indicates a mortality of 15-25 % which many argue is not directly related to procedure but to the general patient debility. This however must be included in the consent as well as the risks of infection, bleeding organ injury and leakage both peritubular or intraperitoneal, aspiration pneumonia.

8. Post operative

Care is taken to ensure the secure fixation of the gastrostomy tubes and the correct intragastric positioning. Should there be any doubt, feeding is interrupted and the position can be rapidly checked by another contrast study. Tube dressings are verified daily and if in doubt as to the patency and position they can be verified specially in restless patients. Nursing the patients in the semi- sitting position may prevent pneumonia in these debilitated patients.

9. Complications

The main complications of Gastrostomy tube placement are:

EARLY

1. Misplacement.
   Using the verification steps as described should prevent any inadvertent placement of the tubes. Before feeding the intragastric position and absence of leakage must be confirmed preferably by a contrast study.
2. Leakage
   This is a troublesome complication and can be prevented and treated by judicious choice of the size othe tube which should be a snug fit. However, in malnourished patients wit severe hypoalbuminemia, the gastrotomy sites can break down, hence the attention paid to insert a wide double purse string.
3. Infection
   Infection of the stoma site can be treated with Metronidazole ointment and daily dressings.
4. Peristomal skin irritation.
   This is due to leakage of acid stomach contents. A barrier dressing of Duoderm is helpful in shielding the skin from the inevitable spillage.

LATE

Later complications include tube slippage, patient pulling the tube out or inadvertent displacement. Once a track has been established, it is a simple matter of replacing the tube with a similar size and type. Once this is achieved, a new contrast study is mandatory to confirm the intragastric position and absence of leakage before resuming feeds.

MORTALITY

The mortality has been described as varying up to 12% (Ref6).

10. References

[1] Nah SA, Narayanaswamy B, Eaton S, Coppi PD, Kiely EM, Curry JI, Drake DP, Barnacle AM, Roebuck DJ, Pierro A. Gastrostomy insertion in children : Percutaneous endoscopic or Percutaneous image guided? J Pediatr Surg. 2010 Jun; 45(6): 1153-8. Fewer PEG patients (28%) had complications than did IG (47%) (P = .001)

[2] Gossage JA, Cho A, Ng PC Technique. Ann R Coll Surg Engl. 2007 Jul; 89(5): 530

[3] Ng PC Single-puncture laparoscopic-assisted gastrostomy. J Laparoendosc Adv Surg Tech A. 1997 Jun; 7(3): 173-5. PMID: 9448129Ng PC

[4] Laparoscopic gastrostomy: a simple way to feed. Surg Laparosc Endosc. 1994 Dec; 4(6): 463-4. PMID:7866620

[5] R. Durai, P. C. H. Ng Simple Technique of Selecting the Correct Feeding Gastrostomy Button. Acta Chir Belg, 2011, **111**, 000-000

[6] Pruthi D, Duerksen DR, Singh H. The practice of gastrostomy tube placement across a Canadian regional health authority. Am J Gastroenterol. 2010 Jul;105(7):1541-50. Epub 2010 Jan 26.

7

Video-Assisted Gastrostomy in Children

Torbjörn Backman, Malin Mellberg, Helén Sjöwie,
Magnus Anderberg and Einar Arnbjörnsson
*Department of Pediatric Surgery, Skåne University Hospital, Lund and Lund University
Sweden*

1. Introduction

A gastrostomy is frequently used as an alternative to a nasogastric tube in children who are unable to manage normal oral feeding for a long time and in whom the nasogastric tube causes respiratory or other problems. Gastrostomy tube placement is associated with frequent postoperative complications and considerable help from the emergency department and outpatient clinic is required for children with gastrostomy tubes.

The history of gastrostomy, from the first known publications through its surgical evolution, is thoroughly described in a previous publication (Gauderer & Stellato, 1986). This work summarizes the different operative procedures that have been described for operatively performing a gastrostomy. These include the time-honored open surgical methods and the more recently introduced minimal invasive methods for gastrostomy. The publication ended with the introduction in 1979 of the percutaneous endoscopic gastrostomy (PEG) procedure (Gauderer et al., 1980). It has been named the world's first natural orifice trans-luminal endoscopic surgery (NOTES). The video-assisted or laparoscopic technique, that was developed before 1990 and entered the scene on a broad scale after 1990, has since then become firmly established and is still widely used.

The PEG method is cheap, fast, and easy to perform but has serious flaws. A shortcoming with the method is that it does not take into account the consequences of the blind puncture through the abdominal cavity and hampers the safety of the child subjected to an operative intervention for a gastrostomy button placement. The serious complications with the PEG procedures in children are well documented and are mainly related to the blind puncture of the abdominal wall (Gauderer, 1991, 2001; Khattak el al, 1998; Kimber et al., 1998; Lantz et al., 2009, 2010) with a risk of perforation of internal organs, bleeding, obstruction or development of a gastroenteric fistula in up to 3.5% (Lantz et al., 2009, 2010; Patwardhan, 2004) of the children.

In order to avoid the complications associated with PEG, the laparoscopy or video-assisted gastrostomy (VAG) technique was developed and used since soon after 1990 (Anderson et al., 1997; Mikaelsson et al., 1995). Laparoscopy reduces the risk of unnoticed intra-abdominal injury and allows for the exact positioning of the gastrostomy site on the stomach as well as on the abdominal wall. Suture of the stomach to the anterior abdominal wall decreases the risk of dislodgement. Placement of a primary low profile gastrostomy button eliminates the need for anesthesia later when changing the gastrostomy device used when performing the PEG technique. The VAG technique may be more technically demanding but is mastered by surgeons today. Furthermore, the VAG technique is more time consuming and may be more expensive. The safety of the children is well worth more time and cost. With time, evidence of the greater safety of the video-assisted technique as compared with the PEG technique has been repeatedly proved and collected in reports (Lantz et al., 2009, 2010) Table 1. Laparoscopy-aided gastrostomy has been found to be a significantly safer procedure than PEG (Aprahamian et al., 2006; Fanelli & Ponsky, 1992; Jones et al., 2007; Kellnar et al., 1999; Rothenberg el al., 1999; Tomicic el al., 2002; Zanakhshary el al., 2005;).

	Percutaneous Endoscopic Gastrostomy PEG	Video-Assisted Gastrostomy VAG	Statistics Method: Fisher's Exact Test
Number of children reported, n = 3441	2599	842	
Number of gastrointestinal complications	40 (1.54%)	0	$p < 0.001$
Number of publications, total: 48, and four publications reported both PEG and VAG	28	16	

Table 1. A summary of the reports in the literature describing complications after minimally invasive gastrostomy in children using Percutaneous Endoscopic Gastrostomy (PEG) or Video-Assisted Gastrostomy (VAG) or laparoscopic gastrostomy. Abstract presented in EUPSA + BAPS Common Congress in Graz, Austria in 17-20 June 2009 (Lantz et al., 2009)

1.1 Indications

The indications for a gastrostomy are nutritional problems in severely ill or neurologically impaired children. Gastrostomy feeding is advocated if nasogastric feeding is likely to persist for more than 6 months (Behrens et al., 1997; Norton et al., 1996). The operation should be carried out only when it is considered that the child's condition would safely allow surgical intervention and when the need for nutritional support is considered necessary for more than 6 months. The VAG procedure is not performed prophylactically.

1.2. Work up

The work up includes an upper GI X- ray to rule out gastric outlet obstruction, hiatal hernia or some gastro-intestinal anomalies. A gastric emptying scan can reveal any gastric emptying problem. All patients should be clinically evaluated for gastro esophageal reflux disease (GERD) before the gastrostomy placement. An endoscopy and 24 h pH measurements should be performed whenever considered necessary. Impedance measurement can be considered especially in younger children with no acid gastro esophageal reflux, in order to evaluate the volume of vomiting and regurgitation into the esophagus and to rule out the indications for surgery for GER.

Gastrostomy operations may be performed on children without being influenced by the child's state of nutrition. This has been motivated by the idea that a gastrostomy would enable fast and secure improvement in the state of nutrition. However, since there is a report on a significant correlation between the child's state of nutrition and the postoperative complications during the first six postoperative months, a routine of nutritional evaluation and support through a nasogastric tube should be considered prior to performing a gastrostomy operation (Backman et al., 2009).

2. The method

The method now used is described here (Backman et al., 2010).

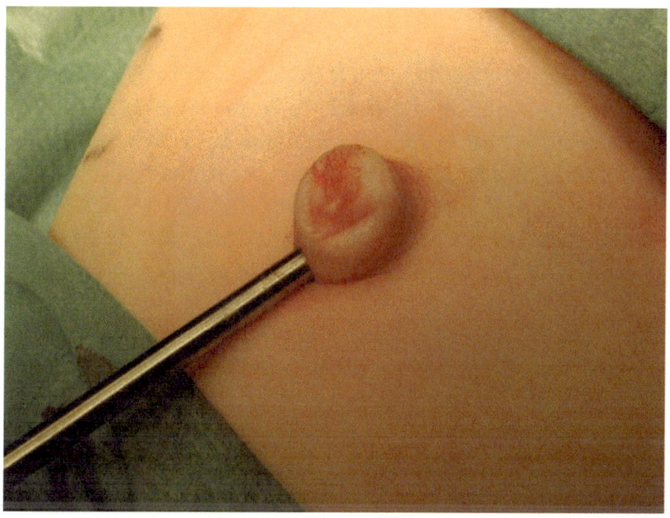

Fig. 1. Two, three or five millimeters trocar is introduced by a mini laparotomy through the umbilicus

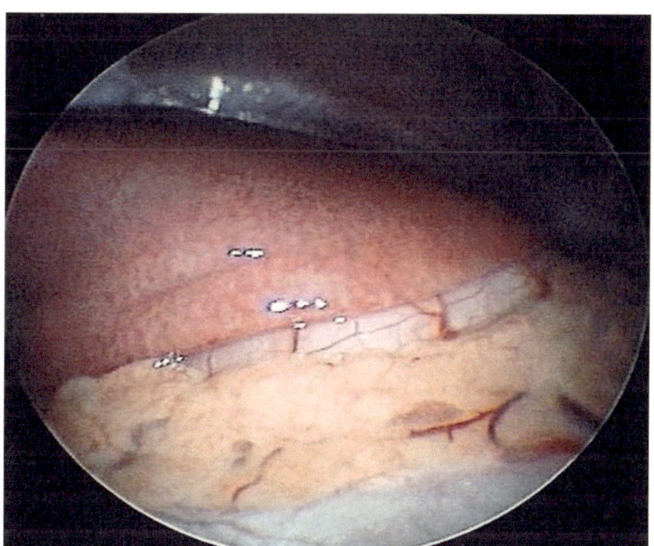

Fig. 2. The stomach is seen under the liver

Prophylactic antibiotics were given prior the operative intervention. All operations were performed under general and local anesthesia. The method of VAG is described in several variations (Mikaelsson et al., 1995; Mikaelsson & Arnbjörnsson, 1998). A 2 to 5 mm trocar is inserted by performing a mini laparotomy through the umbilicus, Figure 1. The abdomen is insufflated with CO_2 up to a pressure of 8 - 10 mmHg at a flow rate of 0.5 - 1.5 l / min. In order to visualize the abdominal cavity a 2 to 5 mm, 0 ° or 30 ° laparoscope optic is used, Figures 2 and 3.
A site for the gastrostomy is chosen approximately at the midpoint from the left costal margin to the umbilicus, through the left rectus muscle, and far enough from the costal margin to ensure that the button does not ride against cartilage when the abdomen is desufflated. At that site, a single 5 mm trocar is placed. Through the trocar, a grasper is passed and used under direct vision to catch the stomach wall at the site selected for the gastrostoma, Figure 4. The grasping site needs to be far enough away from the pylorus to prevent gastric outlet obstruction by the intraluminal balloon on the button, especially in small infants. The stomach wall is then exteriorized when the trocar and the instrument are withdrawn, Figures 5 and 6. If necessary, a clamp is used to mildly dilate the tract. In patients with a thicker abdominal wall, this procedure may be more difficult and the incision may have to be enlarged to allow adequate access to the stomach.

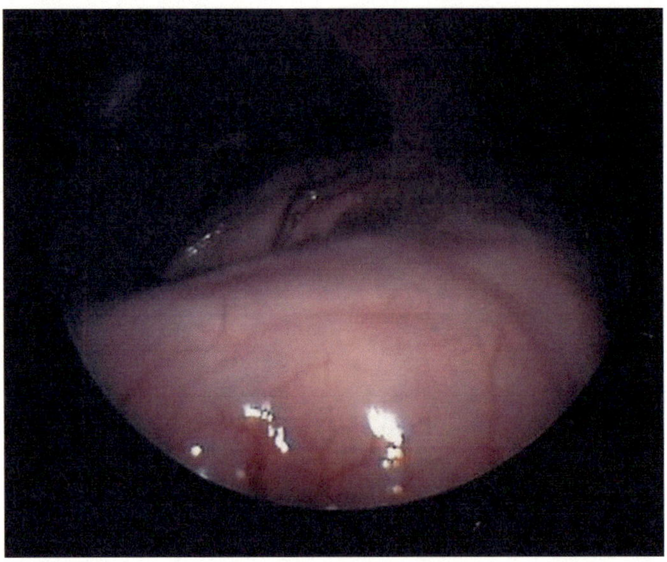

Fig. 3. When the liver is lifted up the stomach is visualized

With the grasper holding the stomach wall, a needle with an absorbable suture is inserted through the abdominal wall, beginning through a small incision half a centimeter from the gastrostoma, Figure 7. The suture is passed through the abdominal wall and then the anterior wall of the stomach and visualized using either the video-scope or under direct vision on the abdominal wall. The suture is then pulled up through the abdominal wall on the contra lateral side half a centimeter from the gastrostoma. The needle is then turned 180 degrees and the procedure repeated, passing the suture back through the two small incisions on each side of the gastrostoma and the stomach, Figure 8. Thus, the stomach is fixated to the abdominal wall with two continuous double U-stitches forming a purse string suture on the stomach wall around the gastrostoma in the center of the loop. To facilitate placement of this suture, the retracted stomach is returned into the abdomen to allow greater exposure of the fascia. It is important not to tighten these sutures until the button is in place, since they pull the stomach back into the abdomen and close the gastrostomy.

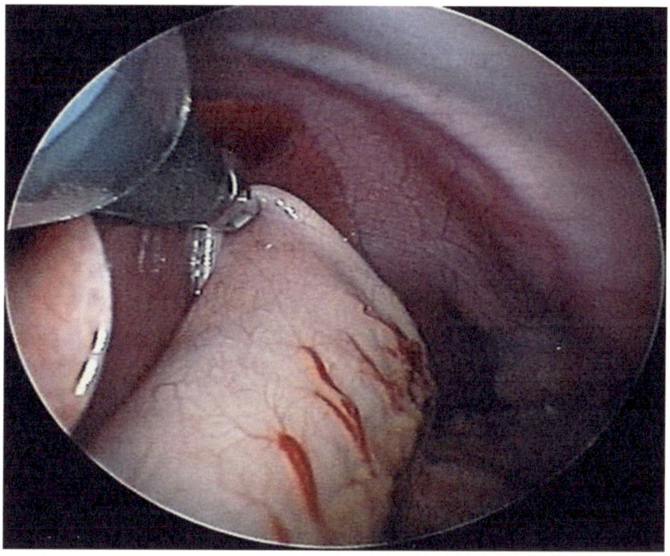

Fig. 4. Where the operating surgeon decides to place the gastrostomy on the stomach the latter is grasped with a two, three or five millimeter grasper through a trocar placed through the abdominal wall where the surgeons decide to place the gastrostomy

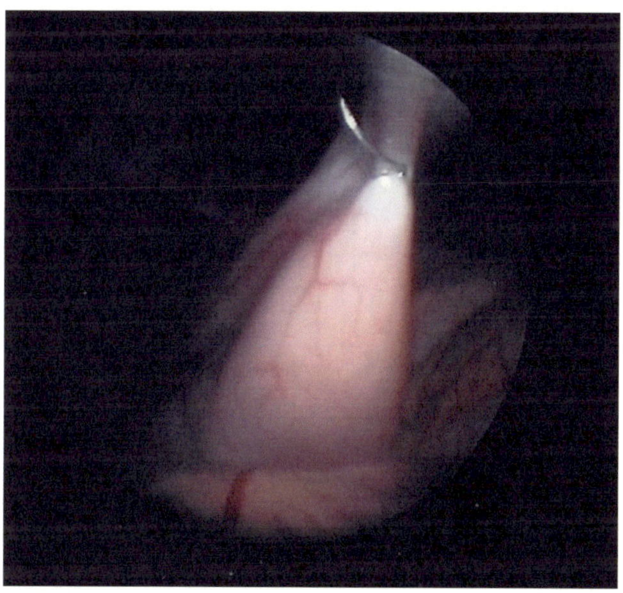

Fig. 5. The stomach wall is grasped and pulled out through the hole in the abdominal wall left when the trocar is withdrawn

After the stitches are placed, the stomach is opened with a needle diathermy or scissors and a catheter inserted, leading the button into the stomach. After measurement, an appropriately sized button (12 - 14 French 1.0- 2.0 cm) with a balloon tip is then placed through the gastrostomy. We use mainly a MicKey® gastrostomy button type (provided by Ballard Medical Product, Draper, UT, USA) or the Mini ONE™ (provided by Applied Medical Technology Inc, Breckville, OH, USA). Lubrication of the button with water may be needed to ease its placement, as the tract is usually quite snug. The suture is tightly tied and the balloon inflated with three to five cc of water. The incision is usually not sutured around the button.

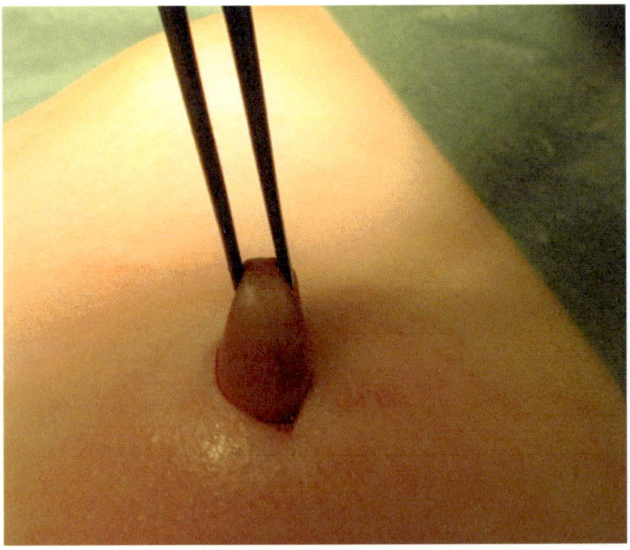

Fig. 6. The stomach wall sticking out through the abdominal wall

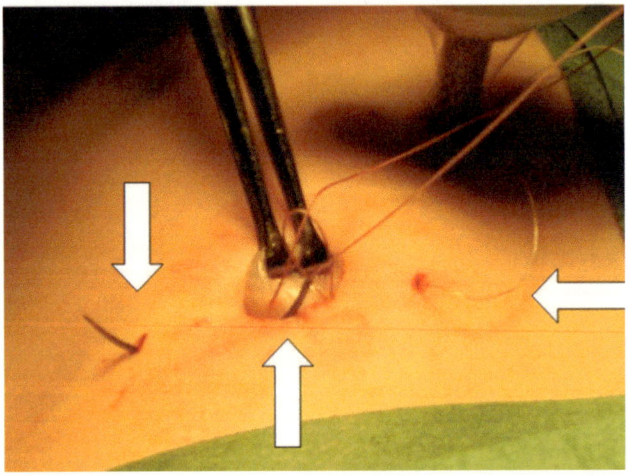

Fig. 7. A photo showing the trocar for the laparoscopy optic in the background and the right arrow pointing to the entrance for the U-stitch suture. The stomach exteriorized and held by graspers indicated by the arrow in the middle and the needle used for the suturing is sticking out as pointed out by the left arrow

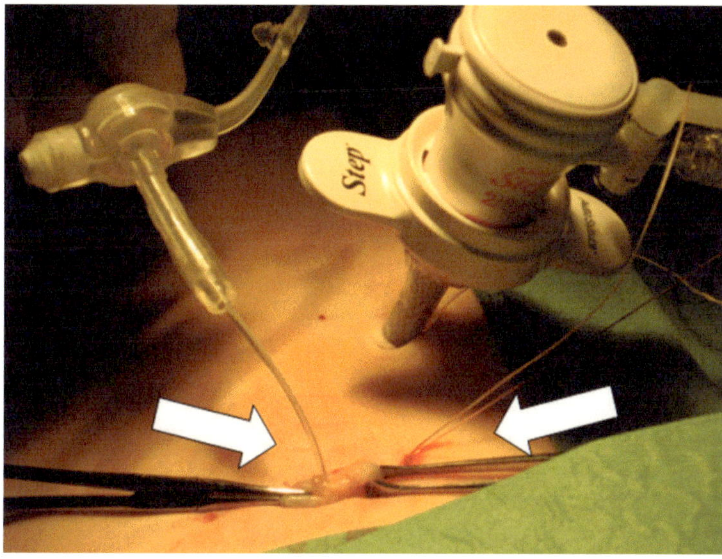

Fig. 8. The double U-stitch suture that forms a purse-string suture around the gastro stoma on the stomach, emerges from the abdomen at the place indicated by the right arrow. The left arrow indicates the stomach, which has been opened and a thin catheter has been inserted and used as a guide for the insertion of the gastrostomy button

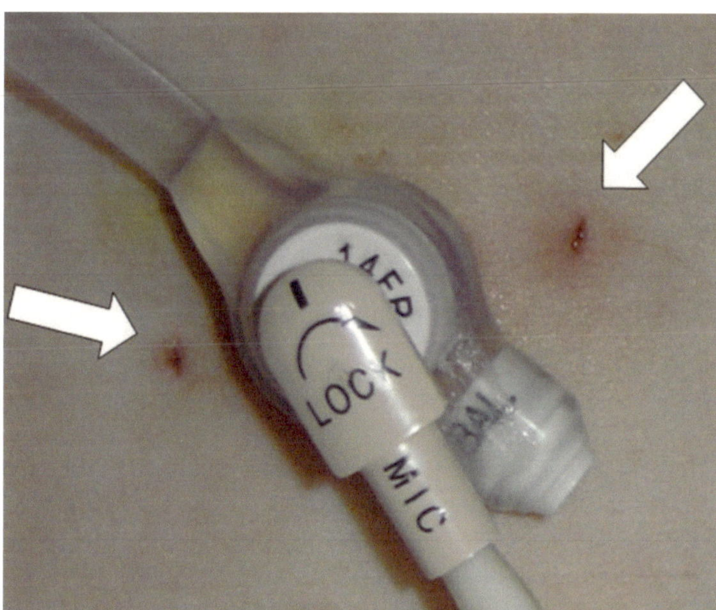

Fig. 9. The gastrostomy button in place. The arrows indicate the locations of the double U-stitch suture

The gastrostomy button in place is shown in Figure 9. On each side of the button two small wounds can be seen. These are the places of the double U-stitch holding the button in place

and forming a purse string suture around the button and the gastro stoma on the stomach. A gastroscopy is performed as the last part of the operative intervention. The view from the stomach through the gastroscopy is shown on Figure 10. The gastroscopy can verify the placement of the gastrostomy button and disclose any anomaly such as hiatal hernia or esophagitis.
Oral feeding is started as soon as the child is awake. Nutrition through the gastrostomy is usually started within 4 hours and continued with increasing amounts of fluid, as tolerated by the child. Bolus or continuous feeding is continued as preoperatively. When it is no longer needed, the gastrostomy button can be removed. We recommend a routine expectance after the removal of a gastrostomy device for at least 1 month. If no spontaneous closure occurs a gastroraphy should be performed (Arnbjörnsson et al., 2005).

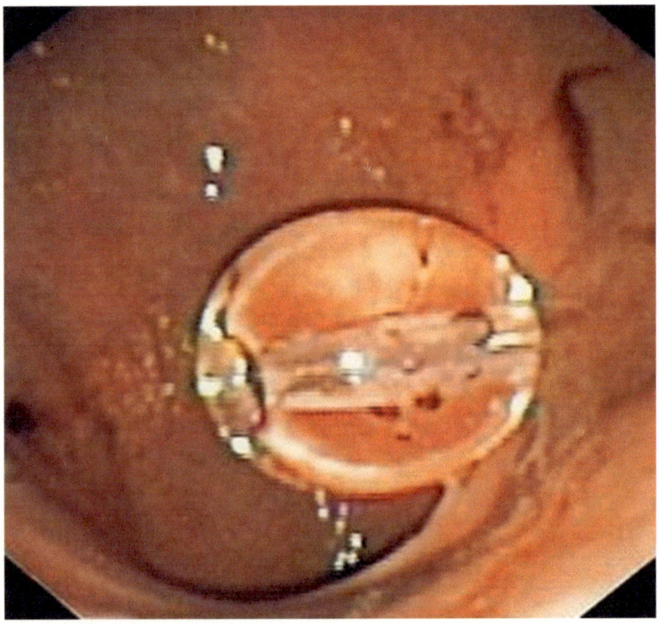

Fig. 10. A view from the gastroscopy showing the balloon on the tip of the gastrostomy button

3. Children

A prospective study was conducted on a heterogeneous group of children who underwent gastrostomy tube placement from June 2006 through February 2011 at a tertiary center for pediatric surgery. The children's comorbidities, Table 2 and demographics, Table 3 are summarized. The children's BMI (Body mass index) is demonstrated in Figure 11.

3.1 Follow-up

The endpoint of the study was six months after the surgery reached by 125 children. All the patients had contact with a dietician and all were prospectively followed up by specially trained nurses during the first postoperative days in hospital and at one and six months after the operation. Additional follow-ups were performed at any time at the request of the child's guardians. All postoperative complications were documented according to a standardized protocol including only those requiring treatment. The registered postoperative complications requiring treatment included:

Severe complications:

- Complications demand emergency re-operations, including bleeding, gastrointestinal fistula or intestinal obstruction.

Minor complications:

- Infectious complications treated with antibiotics and frequent changes of dressing of the wound.
- Granuloma resulting in intervention, such as cauterization or operative intervention.
- Leakage, that required further management, including a change to a new button with a different length or size, or a change of volume in the balloon of the button, or frequent, greater than two times a day, change of dressings.
- Pain around the gastrostoma after the first two postoperative days, treated with analgesics.
- Any discomfort leading to the change of device in the gastrostomy.
- The number of parents' consultations for the child's gastrostomy.

Diagnosis in 135 children	Number of children
Cerebral pares	43 (32%)
Cardiac malformation	25 (19%)
Epilepsy	21 (16%)
Metabolic diseases	18 (13%)
Syndrome	14 (10%)
Cerebral anomaly	12 (9%)
Malformations of the gastrointestinal tract	11 (8%)
Malignancy	8 (6%)
Respiratory insufficiency	7 (5%)
Ventricular - peritoneal shunt	5 (4%)
Mitochondrial disease	4 (3%)
Myopathia	3 (2%)

Table 2. The diagnosis and comorbidity of the included group of 135 children

Age in years	MEAN ± STD	3 ± 3
N = 135	Median (range)	2 (1 month - 14 years)
Weight in kg	MEAN ± STD	11.4 ± 7.6
	Median (range)	9.2 (3.7 – 41)
SD*	MEAN ± STD	- 2.2 ± 1.7
	Median (range)	- 2.1 (-7.1 – 1.3))
Length i cm	MEAN ± STD	82.4 ± 24.4
	Median (range)	78 (36.2 - 162)
SD*	MEAN ± STD	- 1.8 ± 1.7
	Median (range)	- 1.7 (-7.4 – 1.5)
BMI (kg/m^2)	MEAN ± STD	16 ± 2
	Median (range)	15 (11 - 22)

*The individual weight and length at the time of the VAG procedure are shown and assessed by using charts for gender- and age-matched growth standard deviation (SD) scores for Swedish children. Age was approximated to age in months, and weight scores were approximated to the closest whole number in standard deviation. These figures are expressed as weight-for-age Z-scores calculated as: (actual weight-mean weight)/standard deviation (Liou et al., 2001), according to the nationally standardized weight curves (Albertsson-Wikland & Karlberg, 1994).

Table 3. The demography of the children included in the study

4. Results

One hundred and thirty five patients underwent laparoscopic-assisted gastrostomy with the double U-stitch technique and were prospectively evaluated. Three children died from their underlying disease, two after five weeks and one after six months. There were no major complications as bleeding or enteric fistulas requiring emergency reoperations. One hundred and twenty five children reached the endpoint of the study and had been followed for at least six months and were thus included in the report of the results.

Granulation tissue was the most common postoperative complication, occurring in 24% of patients. Two out of three of the patients with granulation tissue had full resolution by the sixth postoperative month, Table 4. At six months postoperatively, a granuloma had developed in 11% of those without any previous granuloma, Table 5. Infection and leakage were also common. Both these minor complications decreased in frequency with time. However, even after six months none of the most usual minor complications disappeared completely. Tube dislodgement was an uncommon complication, occurring 13 times in 125 patients (10%) and resulting in emergency department visits for replacement of the gastrostomy button under general anesthesia in 5 children less than two weeks after the gastrostomy operation, Table 4.

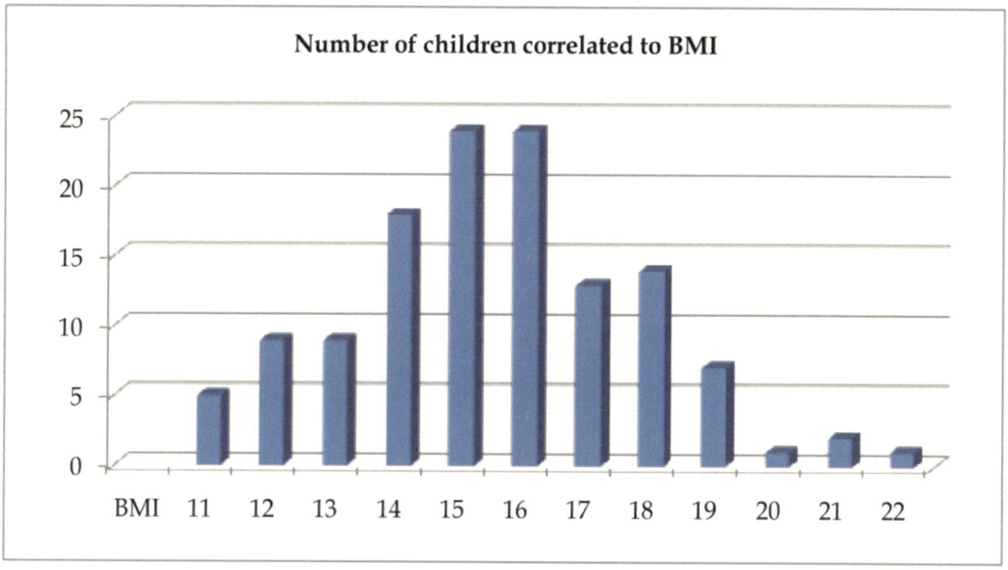

Fig. 11. The summary of the Body mass index (BMI) of the children included in the report

Minor complications	After:		Statistical method: Fisher´s exact test
n = 125	1 month	6 months	p value*
Granuloma	30 (24%)	20 (16%)	0.0365
Vomiting	29 (23%)	20 (16%)	0.2022
Infection	26 (21%)	3 (2%)	<0.0001
treated with antibiotics	20 (16%)	1 (1%)	<0,0001
Leakage	18 (14%)	4 (3%)	0,0012
Tube dislodgement	6 (5%)	7 (6%)	1

Table 4. A summary of the minor complications found at prospective follow-up in 125 out of the 135 children included

A summary of the frequency of minor complications after a video-assisted gastrostomy operation from the perspective of their fate over time is shown in Table 5. A minor complication was not always present directly postoperatively. It could occur later in the progression of the patient. This suggests that the minor complications were not only due to the insertion of the gastrostomy button, but were partly due to the child´s clinical situation during the course of their underlying disease.

Vomiting was an exception to the rule that the minor complications reduced in frequency with time Table 6. The gastrostomy operation does not significantly influence the vomiting which probably depends on the underlying disease and its progress as well as the child´s clinical situation.

Minor complications	After:		Statistical method: CHI2 TEST
N = 125	1 month	6 months	p value
Granuloma	30	10 (33%)	
- No granuloma	95	10 (11%)	< 0.0001
Infection	26	1	
- No infection	99	2	< 0.0001
Leakage	18	1	
- No leakage	102	3	< 0.0001

Table 5. Summary of the frequency of minor complications after a video-assisted gastrostomy operation from the perspective of their fate over time

Vomiting:					
Preoperatively		Postoperatively, after 6 months:			Statistical method: Mann-Whitney U test
N=125		Not vomiting	Kept on vomiting	Started vomiting	P value
Yes	29 (23%)	16 (55%)	13 (45%)	0	
No	96	89 (93%)	0	7 (7%)	0.6650

Table 6. The pre- and postoperative frequency of vomiting in patients undergoing a video-assisted gastrostomy operation

The described method used for the operation is easier the smaller the child and the thinner the abdominal wall. Therefore it was of interest to compare the infants, less than two years of age, with those who were older, with respect to postoperative complications. This comparison is summarized in Table 7 disclosing no practical differences and not suggesting that infants are less prone to postoperative complications, despite the surgeons' impression that the operative intervention is easier with these small patients.

5. Discussion

The primary laparoscopic placement of gastrostomy buttons for feeding tubes is a safe and simple technique and the preferred method of gastrostomy in children (Aprahamian et al., 2006; Fanelli & Ponsky, 1992; Jones et al., 2007; Kellnar et al., 1999; Rothenberg el al., 1999; Tomicic el al., 2002; Zanakhshary el al., 2005;). However, the results show that gastrostomy

tube placement is associated with many early and late complications as has been reported (Arnbjornsson et al., 1999).
The complication rates with VAG in pediatric patients are reported and the subgroups of children who run the highest risk for postoperative complications have been identified. No major complications, defined as life-threatening, have so far been reported in children operated on with VAG. Minor problems including leakage, irritation, and granuloma formation were frequently noted and need care (Arnbjörnsson et al, 1998, 1999; Arnbjörnsson & Larsson, 2005; Backman et al, 2007).

5.1 The treatment of minor complications

In order to avoid the minor problems appearing postoperatively after the placement of a gastrostomy button the following measures can be taken:

- Increase the length of the gastrostomy canal by increasing the distance between two purse string sutures on the stomach wall.
- Wash the skin around the gastrostoma with chlorhexidine (Hibiscrub®) daily during the first five postoperative days.
- Reduce the movements of the gastrostomy button by leaving the feeding catheter in place and fastening it with tape onto the skin during the first five postoperative days.
- The gastrostomy button dimension has been studied and led to the conclusion that a reduction of postoperative gastrostomy site leakage may be gained with the use of gastrostomy buttons of a smaller dimension (Sjövie et al, 2010).

Solid scientific support for the most of these measures is still missing from the literature.

Minor complications	Children's age groups				Statistical method: Fisher´s exact test
n = 125	< 2 years, n = 78		>2 years, n = 47		
Age in years, MEAN ± STD	1 ± 1		6 ± 4		
MEDIAN (range)	1 (0 - 2)		5 (2 - 14)		
Weight in kg, MEAN ± STD	8 ± 3		20 ± 9		
MEDIAN (range)	8 (2 - 14)		16 (9 - 42)		
Number of:	After		After		p value after:
	1 month	6 months	1 month	6 months	1 month/6 months
Granuloma	22	12	8	8	0.0649/0.1909
Vomiting	22	14	7	6	0.0415*/0.1536
Infection	14	2	12	1	0.1069/0.4442
Leakage	12	2	6	2	0.1945/0.3350

*The difference is not statistically significant when using the chi square test or Pearson´s test.

Table 7. Comparison of the number of minor postoperative complications between infants, < 2 years, and older children

5.2 The preoperative state of nutrition

Gastrostomy operations have been performed on children referred to the pediatric surgical clinic without any regard taken to the results of the routine evaluation of the nutritional status of the patient. This has been motivated by the idea that a gastrostomy would enable a fast and secure improvement of the patient in this regard. The question arises whether an improvement in the preoperative nutritional status would reduce the number of

postoperative complications. In a prospective registration (Backman et al., 2009) the nutritional parameters before a gastrostomy operation in a heterogeneous sample of 50 children with nutritional problems were collected. The children were followed up according to a protocol and the occurrence of postoperative complications was correlated to their nutritional status at operation. The hypothesis was that the better the patients' preoperative nutritional status, the fewer the postoperative complications. The aim was to collect information that can be used to improve the practice when performing gastrostomy operations in children, thus increasing the quality of the work as well as improving safety when performing a gastrostomy operation in cases where it is needed.
The routine preoperative evaluation of the children's nutritional status included laboratory tests, as well as weight and length. The age-adjusted Z-score of weight and length to normalize the data relative to a reference population was used. These figures are expressed as weight-for-age Z-scores calculated as: (actual weight-mean weight)/standard deviation (Liou et al., 2001), according to the nationally standardized weight curves (Albertsson-Wikland & Karlberg, 1994). The children were ranked according to the frequency and severity of these postoperative problems up to six months after the gastrostomy operation which was the endpoint of the study. The results disclosed that there was a significant correlation between the frequency of postoperative problems and the low Z-score for weight and length as well as for low phosphate, magnesium and iron levels in the blood at the time of the operation. The results support the necessity of preoperative nutrition evaluation and treatment before a video-assisted gastrostomy operation. These findings are influenced by the fact that the children included had already had a period of treatment and care, and been given a sufficient amount of nutrition through a naso-gastric tube or intravenous nutritional support. The diet anamnesis was intended to be included. However, when this was to be registered, the dietitian had already met the patient and for a while administered the amount of nutrition considered necessary for the child's age and weight. The children under one year of age usually received 100 - 120 kcal/kg/day. The older children received Kcal according to the formula: Kcal/kg/day = 95 - (3 x ages in years), or more when considered necessary. Thus the children's problems were failure to thrive due to complex medical issues and not malnutrition. Therefore, this parameter could not been used. Preoperatively, all the children had had a nasogastric tube for feeding while waiting for the operative intervention to provide the child with a gastrostomy. The latter took place within six weeks from the time when the decision to operate was taken. In spite of this treatment, the difference in the children's nutrition status correlated with the frequency and severity of the postoperative complications. The preoperative intake of nutrition was, in all the patients, considered sufficient for the child's age and weight, and took into account the increased need seen in some patient groups, i.e. children with congenital cardiac anomalies who are in need of up to 40% more nutrition than other children of the same age and weight. Therefore the Z-scores used are not any direct marker of malnutrition, but are more a reflection of a failure to thrive. Postoperatively, no changes were made in the amount of nutrition the child had been given preoperatively.
During the period studied there were no children with tracheostomies. These are well known to have considerable problems with their gastrostomies; the greater effort required to breathe leads to increased abdominal pressure and subsequently more leakage around the gastrostomy tube. The rate of serious complications in this group of patients is lower than that previously reported for PEG or standard Stamm gastrostomies, which is as high as 40% (Rothenberg et al., 1999). The most serious complications were wound infections that,

in this series of patients, were resolved with oral antibiotics or just frequent changes of dressing.

The study revealed a significant correlation between the patients' state of nutrition and the postoperative complications during the first six postoperative months. Thus, the findings bear out a routine of nutritional evaluation and support prior to performing a gastrostomy operation.

5.3 Video-assisted gastrostomy in infants of less than one year of age

The experience with the VAG technique in infants operated on during their first year of life encourages the use of VAG as a safe technique to provide a route for long-term nutritional support even in such young infants (Backman et al, 2005). Aspiration and chest infections, as well as reduction in feeding time and parents' stress are the major reasons for direct enteral feeding using either a nasogastric tube or gastrostomy (Haynes L et al., 1996; Heine et al., 1995).The gastrostomy feeding regimen provides adequate nutrition to promote normal growth and development and supports the increased or special requirements for those patients with an underlying disease condition.

To analyze the nutritional consequences of gastrostomy in infants operated on during their first year of life, an age-adjusted Z-score (Albertsson-Wikland & Karlberg, 1994) was used to normalize the data in relation to a reference population. The body weight was recorded on the day before the operation and at follow-up 6 months later. The weights at operation and at follow-up were compared using the age-adjusted Z-score of weight as describes in the text in Table 3. No corrections were made for prematurity. If the Z-score of weight after operation is higher than before, it indicates an accelerated weight gain i.e. catch-up. The study (Backman et al, 2005) comprised a consecutive series of 53 severely disabled infants aged six months, varying from three weeks to 11 months, who underwent a video-assisted gastrostomy and were prospectively followed up. Included were infants with neurological dysfunction, chromosomal anomalies, metabolic disorders, cardiac anomalies or respiratory insufficiency.

The infants were followed with a scheduled control at 1 and 6 months postoperatively, documenting complications and weight gain. The main outcome measure was the number and type of complications as well as weight gain using the age-adjusted Z-score of weight to normalize the data relative to a reference population. The Z-score increased significantly, illustrating the postoperative weight gain and catch-up. Short- and long-term complications included minor local wound infection, leakage around the gastrostomy tube and granuloma, but none of these were severe.

The results encourage the use of video-assisted gastrostomy as a safe technique to provide a route for long-term nutritional support even in infants less than one year of age. The present study did not reveal any difference between infants less than two years of age, and older children with respect to minor postoperative complications. As in other reports we found an improvement in the patients' nutritional status after supplementary enteral feeding via gastrostomy (Andersson et al., 1997; Chang et al., 2003), in spite of the fact that the children were preoperatively fed by a nasogastric tube. The complication rate was lower than that reported by others in the literature for both PEG and surgical gastrostomy (Gauderer, 1991; Grant, 1988; Haws et al., 1966; Hogan et al., 1986; Kimber et al., 1998; Larson et al., 1987; Marin et al., 1994; Patwardhan et al., 2004). Gastro-colic fistulas, bleeding, leakage to the peritoneal cavity, peritonitis, dislodgement or occlusion of the gastrostomy button were not seen. The problems met by the infants and their parents are scarcely reported in the literature, although they are well known and often seen after a surgical gastrostomy or PEG. These problems, albeit not life-threatening, affect the lives of the infants and their families; they should be taken into account in patient counseling and when discussing the need for a gastrostomy for each individual patient.

The procedure was well tolerated by all the children younger than one year (Backman et al, 2005). No mortality was related to the video-assisted gastrostomy placement. Four infants died of underlying diseases later. Two patients died of intracranial bleeding, one with an astrocytoma and one with a progressive neurological disease. Two died of circulatory failure, one due to a constrictive cardiomyopathy and one due to a cardiac anomaly. There were no deaths related to gastro-oesophageal reflux or pneumonia.

When correlating the incidence of complications in this group of infants (Backman et al, 2005) with different groups of diagnosis, there was no significant difference found between the groups. This is not in agreement with previous reports on 98 children, 0–18 years, where children with congenital heart disease, chronic respiratory failure and metabolic diseases were found to experience the highest rate of minor postoperative complications (Arnbjornsson et al., 1999). Using the method described here as well as the open surgical procedure, the gastrostomy button is put in place directly, eliminating the need for a later change to a gastrostomy button as is the case after a PEG, where this is usually done after 3–6 weeks (Marin et al., 1994). The results encourage the use of video-assisted gastrostomy as a long-term route for safe and effective nutritional support even in children less than one year of age. This is supported by the findings in the present report comparing children younger than two years and those who were older, Table 7.

5.4 Gastro-oesophageal reflux (GER) before and after a video-assisted gastrostomy

Vomiting was a problem before and after a VAG operation in 23% of the children reported here, Table 6. GER has been described as a frequent complication of surgical gastrostomy (Hament et al., 2001; Isch et al., 1997; Launay et al., 1996; Samuel & Holmes, 2002; Doyle & Kennedy 1994; Gottrand & Michaud, 2002). Three prospective studies used 24-h pH monitoring before and after a gastrostomy performed with the percutaneous endoscopic technique (PEG) (Launay et al., 1996; Razeghi et al., 2002; Samuel & Holmes, 2002). In one study (Razeghi et al., 2002) the localization of a PEG-catheter in the antrum of the stomach caused an increase in GER. In an animal study the localization of the gastrostomy to the lesser curvature was associated with a reduced incidence of GER. The ambition was to localize the gastrostomy button at the lesser curvature well above the antrum on the anterior wall of the stomach, thereby reducing the angle of His and increasing the intraabdominal length of the oesophagus (Seekri et al., 1991).

Although gastroesophageal reflux (GER) has been described as a frequent complication of surgical gastrostomy, available data concerning GER and gastrostomy have been conflicting, possibly because of different study designs (Hament et al., 2001; Isch et al., 1997; Launay et al., 1996; Razeghi et al., 2002; Samuel & Holmes, 2002). The risk of developing a gastro esophageal reflux (GER) after a gastrostomy operation is reported. When studying the frequency of GER after VAG the authors concluded that a gastrostomy using the video-assisted technique and placing the stoma on the anterior wall of the stomach close to the lesser curvature does not cause aggravation of acid reflux (Plantin et al, 2006). The question of whether the addition of an antireflux procedure to the gastrostomy might promote better weight gain than a gastrostomy alone remains to be answered. A conclusive comparison is lacking. Theoretically, an antireflux operation should lead to an increase in weight by reducing the losses of energy by vomiting the food. An antireflux operation was not performed in any of the children included in this study at the time it was performed. Vomiting was not a great concern and could be coped with by continuous feeding or frequent feeding with smaller meals. Furthermore, the children's gastroesophageal reflux problems, such as vomiting, disappeared with time and after successful reconstructive cardiac surgery in children with congenital cardiac anomalies. In these situations, an antireflux operation would have been unnecessary.

In a prospective uncontrolled study including 23 neurologically disabled children, from 10 months to 15 years of age, all with severe nutritional problems and in need of a gastrostomy, the frequency of GER pre- and postoperatively was studied (Plantin et al., 2006). The children all had a history of clinical GER problems including vomiting, choking and chest infections. A 24-h pH monitoring was used for a quantitative assessment of GER the day before surgery and 12 months (range 7-22 months) postoperatively. Before the preoperative pH investigation the naso-gastric tube was removed. A Synectics 24 antimony electrode and the Digitrapper recording device (Medtronic Functional Diagnostics A/S, Tonsbakken, Denmark) were used for the 24-h pH monitoring. The electrode was placed fluoroscopically two vertebrae above the diaphragm according to ESPGAN criteria (Vandenplas et al., 1993). The reflux index (RI) was calculated as the percentage of time with pH below 4.

The gastrostomy was placed on the anterior wall of the stomach near the lesser curvature. The main outcome measure was the comparison of the pre- and postoperative 24-h pH monitoring and the reflux index (RI), i.e. the percentage of time with pH below 4. The results showed a no significant reduction of RI from 6.8±4.5 preoperatively to 3.7±2.0 postoperatively. The authors conclude that a gastrostomy using the video-assisted technique and placing the stoma on the anterior wall of the stomach close to the lesser curvature does not cause aggravation of acid reflux. During the observation period the RI decreased in 19 patients and increased in 4. Preoperative gastroscopy disclosed macroscopic oesophagitis in 10 of 23 patients whereas postoperative (7-22 months later) endoscopy performed in 21 patients showed macroscopic signs of oesophagitis in only 3. Two children were later operated on with a fundoplication due to a GER. All the patients had clinical symptoms of GER preoperatively. Two had been treated medically during a short period of 2-4 months postoperatively and at follow-up 12 months (range 7-22 months) later all the patients showed a gain in weight (from 0.6 to 3.8 kg) and regression of clinical reflux symptoms.

The slight decrease in RI in the patient group may be explained not only by the beneficial effect of the gastrostomy technique but also by physiological improvement over time. The decrease in reflux symptoms registered in the group of neurologically disabled patients could, of course, be explained by the need of these particular patients for enteral nutrition. Preoperatively, this had entailed the use of a naso-gastric tube which may have caused reflux as well as upper respiratory problems. This study does not compare the results of this method with any other technique. The important question whether one surgical approach is superior to the other remains unanswered. There is no reason to believe that the method here described is superior to the open surgical technique from the point of view of the exact placement of the gastrostomy tube. With both methods it is possible to place the tube at the same preferred place on the lesser curvature. On the other hand, using the PEG method the site of placement of the tube cannot be easily decided. In conclusion, the data suggest that there is no significant risk for accentuation of GER after a gastrostomy operation using the laparoscopic technique as described, and that a routine performance of concomitant fundoplication cannot be recommended (Georgeson, 1993).

5.5 Gastrostomy in children with cardiac malformations

Cardiac malformations were found in 19% of the children included in this study, Table 2. This high frequency may be due to the fact that the hospital is a tertiary center for cardiac surgery on children. Malnutrition and failure to thrive is a common and well-known problem in the treatment of children with severe congenital heart disease (Mitchell et al., 1995). Three main factors contribute to malnutrition: insufficient oral intake raised metabolic demands, and malabsorption. Adequate growth improves the success of cardiac surgery and influences postoperative morbidity (Blackburn et al., 1977). Previous studies have shown that children with ventricular septal defects have 140% of normal total energy expenditure and 250% of normal energy expenditure of activity (Ackerman et al., 1998). This indicates that children with congenital heart disease may not be able to meet their elevated energy demands. Continuous nasogastric tube feeding has been successful regarding weight gain in children with congenital heart disease (Vanderhoof et al., 1982). Long-term feeding is, however, associated with several disadvantages, such as repeated tube dislocations, gastroesophageal reflux, esophagitis, aspiration, and impaired development of oromotor feeding skills (Warady et al., 1990; Strologo et al., 1997). Retrospective studies of percutaneous endoscopic gastrostomy in children with congenital heart disease have reported an increase in weight (Hofner el al., 2000; Ciotti el al., 2002).

Children with congenital heart disease are reported to have an increased risk of complications after VAG procedures compared to other subgroups of children operated on with VAG (Norén et al, 2007). The aim of that retrospective study was to study the type and frequency of complications and change in weight after a laparoscopic gastrostomy procedure in 31 children with congenital heart disease, comparing patient groups of children with univentricular and biventricular circulation, and with completed and uncompleted cardiac surgery. The main outcome measures were the body weight changes and postoperative complications during follow-up. The results disclosed that minor stoma-related problems were common in both groups. Two severe complications, dislodgements, requiring an operative intervention occurred in the univentricular circulation group. This, together with our previous results of laparoscopy-aided gastrostomy procedures in 98 children with various diseases with no major complications (Arnbjörnsson el al., 1999) might indicate that children with congenital heart disease are at a higher risk of complications than children with other diseases. This is probably more true for children with univentricular circulation, who most likely are more catabolic and, therefore, at an even higher risk of complications than other children with congenital heart disease. Weight was normal at birth, low at the time of the gastrostomy procedure, and did not catch up completely during the follow-up period of a mean of 20 months. There were no significant differences regarding mean weight gain between the groups with univentricular and biventricular circulation.

Children with congenital heart disease seem to have an increased risk of complications after laparoscopy aided gastrostomy procedures, than other children. The laparoscopy-aided gastrostomy procedure has previously been shown to have a low rate of complications and, therefore, we still recommend it to be the first method of choice for the placement of a gastrostomy in children with congenital heart disease. Although there were no significant differences, growth seemed to be slower in children with univentricular circulation as well as those with uncompleted cardiac surgery. This suggests that the energy expenditure in these children could be higher than previously assumed. Possibly the caloric intake, 140% of normal energy expenditure, is insufficient. Further studies are needed to investigate the true energy expenditure in this group of children with severe congenital heart disease and uncompleted cardiac surgery.

5.6 Gastrostomy in children with malignancies

Nutrition in children with a malignant disease often poses serious problems. 6% of the children included in this study had a malignant disease, Table 2. The malignant disease as well as the intensive chemotherapy may result in malnutrition as it may lead to loss of appetite, food aversions, mucositis, nausea and vomiting (Mathew et al., 1996; Pedersen et al., 1999; Skolin et al., 1997). A nasogastric tube has previously been the standard method for administering enteral nutrition to a child with malignant disease who is unable to eat adequately. Tube feeding is associated with several side effects, especially pain from severe mucositis as well as infection and perforation of the esophagus (Doyle & Kennedy 1994). Parenteral nutrition carries the risk of catheter-related infections, and a lack of enteral nutrition may contribute to the passage of bacteria into the systemic circulation (Christensen et al., 1993). Surgery in children with malignancies has been uncertain regarding the relation to the timing of cytostatic drug treatment, posing several questions. Should cytostatic drugs be withheld during the week before surgery and/or the postoperative days? Is the rate of postoperative complications influenced by the immediate administration of cytostatic drugs, and is it higher than when performed in children with neurological disability?

A study was undertaken to test the hypothesis whether the administration of cytostatic drugs close to surgery in children with malignancies influences the rate of postoperative complications after a VAG procedure (Arnbjornsson et al., 2006). The study group comprised a heterogeneous group of 27 children, aged from 6 months to 18 years, with malignancies treated with cytostatic drugs and a VAG procedure. The control group consisted of 27 neurologically impaired children matched for age, sex and operative procedure, selected from a cohort of 154 patients with neurological disabilities operated on with VAG during the same period. The decision to operate did not depend on the timing of the chemotherapy. In the study group the complications were correlated to the time elapsed from completion of the last preoperative or the first postoperative cytostatic drug treatment. The number of days after finishing the last cytostatic treatment and the performance of the VAG were documented. The number of days after surgery to the start of postoperative treatment with cytostatic drugs was also documented. All complications were documented according to a special protocol and correlated to the time elapsed from the last cytostatic drug treatment before and the time of the first treatment after the operation. Significant postoperative complications requiring treatment were included only, e.g. granuloma resulting in intervention such as cauterization or extirpation, infection requiring antibiotics and external leakage demanding some form of management. The complications in the two groups were compared.

The results disclosed no difference in postoperative complications between the study group and the control group. There was no increase in postoperative complications related either to a shorter interval from the last preoperative treatment with cytostatic drugs or timing of the first postoperative cytostatic drug treatment. There was no correlation between white blood cell count, neutrophil count and platelet count at the time of surgery and the frequency of post-surgery complications. In conclusion, the children with malignant diseases did not have more postoperative complications from the VAG than those with neurological defects. There was no correlation to complications regarding timing of the operation and administration of cytostatic drugs.

Surgical intervention in children with malignancies could potentially be more dangerous and subject to a higher frequency of complications as a consequence of the treatment with cytostatic drugs. It has been speculated that children with malignancies and a gastrostomy often have more problems from their gastrostomy while on treatment with cytostatic drugs. It therefore seemed a reasonable assumption that surgery in a child undergoing treatment with cytostatic drugs would lead to more postoperative complications than in neurologically impaired children. The findings of previous studies do not support this suggestion (Arnbjornsson et al., 1999). The study population receiving chemotherapy was heterogeneous and varied widely in age, from 6 months to 18 years, in the type of disease and in the administered chemotherapy. This is significant. For example, age would have had a major effect on the ability of the child to tolerate chemotherapy. Furthermore, age matching with neurologically impaired children does not negate these problems. These children also vary widely in terms of operative risk and complications. A more logical study would have compared oncology children with and without cytotoxic effects, e.g. bone marrow depression. VAG complications in this study were recorded prospectively and therefore were probably more reliable than retrospective information obtained from other reported series in the medical literature. Complications resulting from the VAG button including local infections and mechanical problems with leakage as well as feeding intolerance with nausea, vomiting and diarrhea were reported (Aquino et al., 1995).

There was no increased frequency of complications in the children receiving cytostatic drugs within a few days before or even within one week after surgery. The same types and frequency of complications were encountered in the control group of disabled children with no malignant disease or cytostatic drug treatment (Arnbjornsson et al., 1999). Moreover, the time of cytostatic drug administration did not significantly change the rate of complications. White blood cell count at the time of the operation would be a better marker of chemotherapy effect than the time from chemotherapy. However, this was not statistically verified in this study. The study revealed no aggravated influence of cytostatic drug treatment on early postoperative problems of VAG. The timing of cytostatic drug administration in relation to the surgical intervention did not influence the frequency of postoperative complications. As a conclusion of the study a VAG procedure was recommended even in children with a malignant disease. A postponement of cytostatic treatment for some days after surgery was suggested despite the lack of clear evidence supporting this statement.

5.7 Gastrostomy in children with ventricular-peritoneal shunt (VPS)

Ventricular-peritoneal shunt (VPS) occurring in 4% of the included children, Table 2, is frequently associated with complications, such as shunt obstruction, infection and migration with or without erosion into nearby structures. These complications may occur at the abdominal site of a VPS raising the question of whether concurrent use of a separate intra-abdominal catheter such as a PEG, is safe and effective. Surgical intervention in children with VPS could potentially be more dangerous and subject to a higher frequency of complications. Many of the complications from VPS could preclude a VAG operation or raise serious concern with respect to VAG placement. Thus, it is acknowledged that the rate of peritonitis may be increased by the presence of a VPS. This issue remains unresolved and is influenced by institutional and individual expertise of which some have concluded that simultaneous placement of a VPS and PEG should be avoided since some 5-10% of all inserted VP shunts eventually require revision for infection (Taylor et al., 2001).

The infective complications of PEG include stoma site infection in 3–9% and peritonitis in 1–7% (Sane et al., 1998). The standard pull-through technique of PEG insertion exposes the gastrostomy tube to oropharyngeal bacterial flora. Thus, following PEG, there are a number of factors that could lead to an intra-peritoneal catheter becoming exposed to bacterial pathogens. This theoretically increased risk for VP shunt infections after PEG insertion has however, not yet been established. On the contrary, previous reports have shown that there was no significant morbidity associated with a PEG in the presence of a VPS (Graham et al., 1993; Baird &, Salasidis, 2004).

The safety of VAG was prospectively studied in children who had a ventriculoperitoneal shunt (VPS) (Backman et al., 2007). The study was undertaken to test the hypothesis whether the presence of a VPS influences the type and frequency of complications after a VAG procedure in children. The study group comprised a heterogeneous sample of 15 consecutive children, aged from 2 months to 12 years, with VPS, operated on with the VAG procedure and prospectively included. The control group consisted of 15 neurologically disabled children without VPS, matched for age, sex and operative procedure, retrospectively selected from a cohort of 167 patients with neurological disabilities operated on with VAG during the study period. All the patients were clinically evaluated for GER before the gastrostomy placement. In nine studied patients and in eight control patients an endoscopy and 24 h pH measurements were performed. None had the indications for surgery for GER. No patient in the present study had clinical signs of an intra-abdominal infection at the time of PEG placement and none were on steroid or cytostatic medication. All the VPS had been placed at least 8 weeks prior to the placement of the gastrostomy button. There were no serious operative complications, such as puncture of hollow organs or bleeding. In the immediate postoperative period, no wound or intra-abdominal complications occurred. There were no reoperations of the VAG due to adhesions or leakage. There was no difference in postoperative complications between the study and the control group.

Although the study does not indicate that children with VPS who undergo the VAG procedure are at greater risk of infection and subsequent shunt malfunction, there are other studies recommending prophylactic antibiotic therapy to cover skin and oral flora (Baird &, Salasidis, 2004; Taylor et al., 2001). The patients in the presented study all received antibiotic prophylaxis. The placement of a percutaneous gastrostomy feeding tube, in the acute phase, in children with brain tumors and VP shunts may increase the risk of ascending meningitis especially if there are early gastrostomy-related complications (Gassas et al., 2006). Greatly disabled patients often have other potential risk factors for VP shunt infections, such as poor nutritional status, long-term hospitalization, subclinical infections and pressure ulcers. There seems to be consensus in the literature that antibiotic prophylaxis for PEG insertion is desirable in order to reduce the percentage of PEG site infection (Nicholson et al, 2000).

Co-placement of PEG and a VPS is reported (Nabika et al., 2006). The authors recommended at least 1 month between the procedures as well as administration of antibiotic prophylaxis. In the case series presented here, there was a lapse of at least 2 months between VPS and VAG. The VAG complications in this study were recorded prospectively and were, therefore, more reliable than retrospective information obtained from other reported series in the medical literature. The complications from the VAG button were recorded, including local infections and mechanical problems with pain and leakage. Contrary to expectations, no increased frequency of complications was found following VAG in the children with VPS. The same types and frequency of complications were encountered in the control group of disabled children with no malignant disease or cytostatic drug treatment as had been reported earlier (Arnbjornsson et al., 2006).

Placement of a gastrostomy button in patients with VPS raises valid concern for CNS infection and shunt malfunction. Thus the gastrostomy button should be put in place several weeks after VPS placement, and the patients should be given an antibiotic prophylactically to prevent infection with skin flora. Using the laparoscopy and visualizing the VPS catheter is preferable to a blind trans-abdominal puncture as when using the PEG technique. The study indicates that children with VPS who undergo a VAG are at no greater risk of infection and subsequent shunt malfunction. Until the results of larger clinical trials are available, it is recommended to use VAG in patients with VPS when long-term enteral nutrition is required. The children with ventricular-peritoneal shunt (VPS) who underwent a VAG button placement were not at high risk for infection and subsequent shunt malfunction. They did not have more postoperative problems than a matched control group of neurologically disabled children (Backman et al, 2007).

5.8 Closure after gastrostomy button removal

A gastrostomy device is removed from the gastrostomy when no longer needed and the stoma usually closes within a short period of time without any surgical measures. Occasionally spontaneous closure does not occur and the stoma has to be closed surgically. For the patient the operative procedure includes a laparotomy and closure of the stomach wall and the abdominal wall in separate layers. The question is whether it is possible for the surgeon to decide which stoma has to be closed with a gastroraphy and which to leave for a spontaneous closure within a reasonable period of time. It would be of importance to find a factor correlating to the spontaneous closure of a gastrostomy after the device or button had been removed from the stoma. This knowledge regarding when to decide which gastrostomy has to be closed surgically and which to leave for spontaneous closure within a short time would be valuable to the surgeon. Gastrostomies constructed by using VAG or PEG are considered equal when it comes to spontaneous closure or the need for a gastroraphy. Although not studied we have no reason to believe that gastrostomy after a PEG would behave otherwise. The resulting gastrostomy has similar anatomical structures and thus it seems logical that a PEG and a VAG behaves similar.

Out of a cohort of 321 patients, who had been operated on with a video-assisted gastrostomy, all the 48 (15%) patients who had their gastrostomy button removed were included. The children were postoperatively carefully followed up and the closure of the gastrostomy was registered. According to the old institutional routine the child waited at least 3 months after the removal of the gastrostomy device before suggesting to the child's guardians an operative closure of the stoma (Arnbjornsson et al., 2005). Spontaneous closure of the gastrostomy happened in 26 patients within a 3-month expectance. In 14 of these 26 children the closure occurred within 2 weeks and in a further six children within 1 month. In only one child did the gastrostomy close spontaneously after 2 months. With the same expectance period the stoma did not close in 22 patients and they were consequently operated on with a gastroraphy. In 13 patients this procedure was performed within 5 weeks.

There was no difference found between the two groups regarding the patients' diagnoses, the duration of the gastrostomy use or the patient's age at the time of removal of the gastrostomy device. The small numbers of patients in each group of diagnosis made statistical calculations insignificant. Thus the hypothesis that any factor could predict the closure of the gastrostomy was consequently rejected. Thus, a routine expectance after the removal of a gastrostomy device for a short time of one month is recommended. If no spontaneous closure occurs, then a gastroraphy should be performed. A randomized study should replace the kind of observations reported here. However, such a randomized study would lead to an unnecessary gastroraphy in some patients or a long waiting time to a gastroraphy in others.

From the surgical point of view it is important that the gastroraphy is performed under general anesthesia. The procedure starts with a circular incision around the gastrostomy and the dissection is performed through the abdominal wall down to the stomach wall without opening the abdomen. We routinely close the stomach wall and the abdominal wall separately. This routine is based on our previous experience of cases where the opening was simply closed by a small local procedure suturing only the skin and subcutaneous tissue without layered closure. In all the patients, the postoperative course was complicated by a subcutaneous leakage from the stomach causing an infection. A third option doing a laparotomy into free abdomen would be too extensive in these cases. Evidence based on a randomized study comparing these methods is still missing.

6. The future

The future will provide better materials and design of the gastrostomy buttons and thereby avoid complications reported to be due to the design of the gastrostomy button (Arnbjörnsson et al., 1998). The materials used in the gastrostomy buttons and feeding tubes are still under development as is the construction of gastrostomy buttons. As technology improves so will its use for the children in need of a gastrostomy. Time will tell if the method described here can be further improved or replaced with still safer and better procedures for the children in need of a gastrostomy.

The way of performing a gastrostomy in children described here is certainly not the only way. Nor is it the definite final solution to the problem of performing a gastrostomy operation in children. Surgeons have been very creative in performing this simple communication between the stomach and the external surface of the body and let us hope that their ingenious talents and inventions will continue to flourish in the future for the benefit of the small patients. The equipment used in surgery today will improve and new technique inventions will enter the scene. The rapid development seen in the surgical field will also lead to new technology in the field of gastrostomies, unknown today.

7. Acknowledgments

We are indebted to Gillian Sjödahl, Lexis English for Writers, Lund, Sweden, for linguistic revision of the manuscript.

8. Ethical considerations

Intention to treat was the main analysis strategy and encompassed all the patients included in the studies reported. The regional research ethics committee approved the studies.

9. Competing interests

When performing this work, there were no external influences or conflicts of interests. All authors declare:

1. No financial support for the submitted work from anyone other than their employer;
2. No financial relationships with commercial entities that might have an interest in the submitted work;
3. No spouses, partners, or children with relationships with commercial entities that might have an interest in the submitted work;
4. No non-financial interests that may be relevant to the submitted work.

10. Legal requirements

This report complies with the current laws of the country in which it was performed.

11. Funding

This study was funded only by the Pediatric Surgical center involved.

12. References

Ackerman, IL; Karn, CA.; Denne, SC.; Ensing, GJ. & Leitch, CA. (1998). Total but not resting energy expenditure is increased in infants with ventricular septal defects. *Pediatrics,* 102:1172–1177

Albertsson-Wikland, K. & Karlberg, J. (1994). Natural growth in children born small for gestational age with and without catchup growth. *Acta Paediatr Suppl* 399:64–70

Andersson, L.; Mikaelsson, C.; Arnbjörnsson, E. & Larsson, LT. (1997). Laparoscopy aided gastrostomy in children. *Ann Chir Gynaecol.* 86:19-22

Aprahamian, CJ.; Morgan, TL.; Harmon, CM.; Georgeson, KE. & Barnhart, DC. (2006). U-stitch laparoscopic gastrostomy technique has a low rate of complications and allows primary button placement: experience with 461 pediatric procedures. *J Laparoendosc Adv Surg Tech A.* 16:643-9

Aquino, VM.; Smyrl, CB.; Hagg, R.; McHard, KM.; Prestridge, L. & Sandler, ES. (1995). Enteral nutritional support by gastrostomy tube in children with cancer. *J Pediatr* 127:58-62

Arnbjornsson, E.; Larsson, LT. & Lindhagen T. (1999). Complications of laparoscopy-aided gastrostomies in pediatric practice. *J Pediatr Surg* 34:1843-1846

Arnbjörnsson, E.; Backman, T.; Berglund, Y. & Kullendorff, CM. (2005). Closure after gastrostomy button. PediatrSurg Int. Oct; 21(10):797-799. Epub 2005 Oct 21

Arnbjörnsson, E.; Backman, T.; Mörse, H.; Berglund Y.; Kullendorff, CM. & Lövkvist, H. (2006). Complications of video-assisted gastrostomy in children with malignancies or neurological diseases. *ActaPaediatr.* Apr; 95(4):467-470

Arnbjörnsson, E.; Jakobsson, I.; Larsson, LT. & Mikaelsson, C. (1998). Gastrostomy button causing perforation of the posterior gastric wall. *ActaPaediatr.* Nov; 87(11):1203-1204

Arnbjörnsson, E. & Larsson, LT. (1998). Laparoscopic button is a safe method in pediatric gastrostomy. *Lakartidningen.* Sep 9; 95(37):3919. Swedish

Arnbjörnsson, E. & Larsson, LT. (2005). Video-assisted placing of a gastrostomy button in children. Ten years of experiences show advantages of the method. *Lakartidningen* Nov 14-20; 102(46):3451-3455. Swedish.

Backman, T.; Arnbjörnsson, E.; Berglund, Y. & Larsson, LT. (2006). Video-assisted gastrostomy in infants less than 1 year. *PediatrSurg Int.* Mar; 22(3):243-246. Epub 2006 Jan 10

Backman, T.; Arnbjörnsson, E. & Kullendorff, CM. (2005). Omentum herniation at a 2-mm trocar site. *J Laparoendosc Adv Surg Tech A.* Feb; 15:87-88

Backman, T.; Berglund, Y.; Sjövie, H. & Arnbjörnsson E. (2007). Complications of video-assisted gastrostomy in children with or without a ventriculoperitoneal shunt. *PediatrSurg Int.* Jul;23(7):665-8. Epub 2007 May 9

Backman, T.; Sjövie, H.; Kullendorff, CM. & Arnbjörnsson, E. (2009). Correlation between the preoperative state of nutrition and the frequency of postoperative problems after video-assisted gastrostomy in children. *Gastroenterology Insights* volume 1:e2

Backman, T.; Sjövie, H.; Kullendorff, CM. & Arnbjörnsson, E. (2010). Continuous double U-stitch gastrostomy in children. *Eur J Pediatr Surg.* Jan;20(1):14-17. Epub 2009 Oct 14

Baird, R. & Salasidis, R. (2004). Percutaneous gastrostomy in patients with a ventriculoperitoneal shunt: case series and review. *Gastrointest Endosc* 59:570–574

Behrens, R.; Lang, T.; Muschweck, H.; Richter, T. & Hofbeck, M. (1997). Percutaneous endoscopic gastrostomy in children and adolescents. *J Pediatr Gastroenterol Nutr.* 25:487–491

Blackburn, GI.; Gibbons, GW.; Bothe, A.; Benotti, PN.; Harken, DE. & McEnany, TM. (1977). Nutritional support in cardiac cachexia. *J Thorac Cardiovasc Surg* 1977; 73:489–496

Chang, PF.; Ni, YH. & Chang, MH. (2003). Percutaneous endoscopic gastrostomy to set up a long-term enteral feeding route in children: an encouraging result. *Pediatr Surg Int* 19:283–285

Christensen, ML.; Hancock, M.; Gattuso, J.; Hurwitz, CA.; Smith, C.; McCormick, J. & Mirro J Jr. (1993). Parenteral nutrition associated with increased infection rate in children with cancer. *Cancer* 72:2732-2738

Ciotti, G.; Holzer, R.; Pozzi, M. & Dalzell, M. (2002). Nutritional support via percutaneous endoscopic gastrostomy in children with cardiac disease experiencing difficulties with feeding. *Cardiol Young* 12:537–541

Doyle, FM. & Kennedy, NP. (1994). Nutritional support via percutaneous endoscopic gastrostomy. *Proc Nutr Soc* 53:473–482

Fanelli, RD. & Ponsky, JL (1992). A simplified technique for percutaneous endoscopic gastrostomy. *Surg Endosc.*6:261–262

Gassas, A.; Kennedy, J.; Green, G.; Connolly, B.; Cohen, J.; Dag-Ellams, U.; Kulkarni, A. & Bouffet, E . (2006). Risk of ventriculoperitoneal shunt infections due to gastrostomy feeding tube insertion in pediatric patients with brain tumors. *Pediatr Neurosurg* 42:95–99

Gauderer, MW.; Ponsky, JL. & Izant, RJ Jr. (1980). Gastrostomy without laparotomy: a percutaneous endoscopic technique. *J Pediatr Surg.* Dec;15(6):872-5

Gauderer, MW. & Stellato, TA. (1986). Gastrostomies: evolution, techniques, indications, and complications. *Curr Probl Surg.* Sep;23(9):657-719

Gauderer, MW. (1991). Percutaneous endoscopic gastrostomy: A 10-year experience with 220 children. *J Pediatr Surg* 26:288–294

Gauderer, MW. (2001). Percutaneous endoscopic gastrostomy-20 years later: a historical perspective. *J Pediatr Surg* 36:217–219

Georgeson, KE. (1993). Laparoscopic gastrostomy and fundoplication. *Pediatr Ann* 22:675–677

Gottrand, F. & Michaud, L. (2002). Percutaneous endoscopic gastrostomy and gastro-esophageal reflux: are we correctly addressing the question? *J Pediatr Gastroenterol Nutr.* 35:22–24

Graham, SM.; Flowers, JL.; Scott, TR.; Lin, F. & Rigamonti, D. (1993). Safety of percutaneous endoscopic gastrostomy in patients with a ventriculoperitoneal shunt. *Neurosurgery* 32:932–934

Grant, JP. (1988). Comparison of percutaneous endoscopic gastrostomy with Stamm gastrostomy. *Ann Surg* 207:598–603

Hament, JM.; Bax, NM.; van der Zee, DC.; De Schryver, JE. & Nesselaar, C. (2001). Complications of percutaneous endoscopic gastrostomy with or without concomitant antireflux surgery in 96 children. *J Pediatr Surg* 36:1412–1415

Haws, EB.; Sieber, WK. & Kiesewetter, WB (1996). Complications of tube gastrostomy in infants and children. 15-year review of 240 cases. *Ann Surg* 164:284–290

Haynes, L.; Atherton, DJ.; Ade-Ajayi, N.; Wheeler, R. & Kiely, EM. (1996). Gastrostomy and growth in dystrophic epidermolysis bullosa. *Br J Dermatol* 134:872–879

Heine, RG.; Reddihough, DS. & Catto-Smith, AG. (1995). Gastrooesophageal reflux and feeding problems after gastrostomy in children with severe neurological impairment. *Dev Med Child Neurol* 37:320–329

Hofner, G.; Behrens, R.; Koch, A.; Singer, H. & Hofbeck, M. (2000). Enteral nutritional support by percutaneous endoscopic gastrostomy in children with congenital heart disease. *Pediatr Cardiol* 21:341–346

Hogan, RB.; DeMarco, DC.; Hamilton, JK.; Walker, CO. & Polter, DE. (1986). Percutaneous endoscopic gastrostomy—to push or pull. A prospective randomized trial. *Gastrointest Endosc* 32:253–258

Isch, JA.; Rescorla, FJ.; Scherer, LR 3rd.; West, KW. & Grosfeld, JL. (1997). The development of gastroesophageal reflux after percutaneous endoscopic gastrostomy. *J Pediatr Surg* 32:321–323

Jones, VS.; La Hei, ER. & Shun, A. (2007). Laparoscopic gastrostomy: the preferred method of gastrostomy in children. *Pediatr Surg Int.* 23:1085-9

Kellnar, ST.; Till, H. & Bohn, R. (1999). Laparoscopically assisted performance of gastrostomy—a simple, safe and minimal invasive technique. *Eur J Pediatr Surg* 9:297–298

Khattak, IU.; Kimber, C.; Kiely, EM. & Spitz, L. (1998). Percutaneous endoscopic gastrostomy in paediatric practice: Complications and outcome. *J Pediatr Surg* 33:67–72

Kimber, CP.; Khattak, IU.; Kiely, EM. & Spitz, L. (1998). Peritonitis following percutaneous gastrostomy in children: management guidelines. *ANZ J Surg* 68:268–270

Lantz, M.; Hultin Larsson, H. & Arnbjörnsson, E. (2010). Literature review comparing laparoscopic and percutaneous endoscopic gastrostomies in a pediatric population. *Int J Pediatr.* 2010:507616. Epub 2010 Mar 10

Lantz, M.; Larsson, HH. & Arnbjörnsson, E. (2009). Video-assisted technique is best when performing laparoscopic gastrostomy in children. Meta-analysis of the frequency of fistulas following two different methods. *Lakartidningen.* Nov 11-17; 106(46):3078, 3080-3082. Swedish

Larson, DE.; Burton, DD.; Schroeder, KW. & DiMagno, EP. (1987). Percutaneous endoscopic gastrostomy. Indications, success, complications, and mortality in 314 consecutive patients. *Gastroenterology* 93:48–52

Launay, V.; Gottrand, F.; Turck, D.; Michaud, L.; Ategbo, S. & Farriaux, JP. (1996). Percutaneous endoscopic gastrostomy in children: influence on gastroesophageal reflux. *Pediatrics* 97:726–728

Liou, TG.; Adler, FR.; Fitzsimmons, SC.; Cahill, BC.; Hibbs, JR. & Marshall, BC. (2001). Predictive 5-year survivorship model of cystic fibrosis. *Am J Epidemiol* 53:345–352

Marin, OE.; Glassman, MS.; Schoen, BT. & Caplan, DB. (1994). Safety and efficacy of percutaneous endoscopic gastrostomy in children. *Am J Gastroenterol* 89:357–361

Mathew, P.; Bowman, L.; Williams, R.; Jones, D.; Rao, B.; Schropp, K.; Warren, B.; Klyce, MK.; Whitington, G. & Hudson, M. (1996). Complications and effectiveness of gastrostomy feedings in pediatric cancer patients. *J Pediatr Hematol Oncol* 18:81-85

Mikaelsson, C.; Arnbjörnsson, E. & Larsson, LT. (1995). The laparoscopy button. A new method with minimal surgical trauma in gastrostomy in children. *Lakartidningen.* Sep 6; 92(36):3237-3238. Swedish

Mikaelsson, C. & Arnbjörnsson, E.(1998). Single-puncture laparoscopic gastrostomy in children. *PediatrSurg Int.* Nov; 14(1-2):43-44

Mitchell, IM.; Logan, RW.; Pollock, JC. & Jamieson, MP. (1995). Nutritional status of children with congenital heart disease. *Br Heart J* 73:277–283

Nabika, S.; Oki, S.; Sumida, M.; Isobe, N.; Kanou, Y. & Watanabe Y. (2006). Analysis of risk factors for infection in coplacement of percutaneous endoscopic gastrostomy and ventriculoperitoneal shunt (discussion 229- 230). *Neurol Med Chir* (Tokyo) 46:226–229

Nicholson, FB.; Korman, MG. & Richardson, MA. (2000). Percutaneous endoscopic gastrostomy: a review of indications, complications and outcome. *J Gastroenterol Hepatol* 15(1):21–25

Norén, E.; Gunnarsdóttir, A.; Hanséus, K. & Arnbjörnsson, E. (2007). Laparoscopic gastrostomy in children with congenital heart disease. *J LaparoendoscAdvSurg Tech A.* Aug; 17(4):483-948

Norton, B.; Homer-Ward, M.; Donnelly, MT.; Long, RG. & Holmes, GK. (1996). A randomised prospective comparison of percutaneous endoscopic gastrostomy and nasogastric tube feeding after acute dysphagic stroke. *BMJ* 312:13–16

Patwardhan, N.; McHugh, K.; Drake, D. & Spitz, L. (2004). Gastroenteric fistula complicating percutaneous endoscopic gastrostomy. *J Pediatr Surg* 39:561–564

Pedersen, AM.; Kok, K.; Petersen, G.; Nielsen, OH.; Michaelsen, KF. & Schmiegelow, K. (1999). Percutaneous endoscopic gastrostomy in children with cancer. *Acta Paediatr* 88:849-852

Plantin, I.; Arnbjörnsson, E. & Larsson, LT. (2006). No increase in gastroesophageal reflux after laparoscopic gastrostomy in children. *Pediatr Surg Int.* Jul; 22(7):581-4. Epub 2006 Jun 1

Razeghi, S.; Lang, T. & Behrens, R. (2002). Influence of percutaneous endoscopic gastrostomy on gastroesophageal reflux: a prospective study in 68 children. *J Pediatr Gastroenterol Nutr* 35:27–30

Rothenberg, SS.; Bealer, JF.; & Chang, JH. (1999). Primary laparoscopic placement of gastrostomy buttons for feeding tubes: A safer and simpler technique. *Surg Endosc* 13:995-997

Samuel, M. & Holmes, K. (2002). Quantitative and qualitative analysis of gastroesophageal reflux after percutaneous endoscopic gastrostomy. *J Pediatr Surg* 37:256-261

Sane, SS.; Towbin, A.; Bergey, EA.; Kaye, RD.;, Fitz, CR.; Albright, L. & Towbin, RB. (1998). Percutaneous gastrostomy tube placement in patients with ventriculoperitoneal shunts. *Pediatr Radiol* 28:521-523

Seekri, IK.; Rescorla, FJ.; Canal, DF.; Zollinger, TW.; Saywell, R Jr. & Grosfeld, JL. (1991). Lesser curvature gastrostomy reduces the incidence of postoperative gastroesophageal reflux. *J Pediatr Surg* 26:982-985

Sjövie, H.; Larsson, LT. & Arnbjörnsson, E. (2010). Postoperative gastrostomy site leakage correlated to the dimension of the gastrostomy button in children. *Gastroenterology Insights* volume 2:e9

Skolin, I.; Axelsson, K.; Ghannad, P.; Hernell, O. & Wahlin, YB. (1997). Nutrient intake and weight development in children during chemotherapy for malignant disease. *Oral Oncol* 33:364-368

Strologo, LD.; Principato, F.; Sinibaldi, D.; Appiani, AC.; Terzi, F.; Dartois, AM. & Rizzoni, G. (1997). Feeding dysfunction in infants with severe chronic renal failure after long-term nasogastric tubefeeding. *Pediatr Nephrol* 11:84-86

Taylor, AL.; Carroll, TA.; Jakubowski, J. & O'Reilly, G. (2001). Percutaneous endoscopic gastrostomy in patients with ventriculoperitoneal shunts. *Br J Surg* 88:724-727

Tomicic, JT.; Luks, FI.; Shalon, L. & Tracy, TF. (2002). Laparoscopic gastrostomy in infants and children. *Eur J Pediatr Surg* 12:107-110

Vandenplas, Y.;Ashkenazi, A.; Belli, D.; Boige, N.; Bouquet, J.; Cadranel, S.; Cezard, JP.; Cucchiara, S.; Dupont, C. & Geboes, K. (1993). A proposition for the diagnosis and treatment of gastro-esophageal reflux disease in children: a report from a working group on gastro-esophageal reflux disease. *Eur J Pediatr* 152:704-711

Vanderhoof, JA.; Hofschire, PJ.; Baluff, MA.; Guest, JE.; Murray, ND.; Pinsky, WW.; Kugler, JD. & Antonson, DL. (1982). Continuous enteral feedings: An important adjunct to the management of complex congenital heart disease. *Am J Dis Child* 136:825-827

Warady, BA.; Kriley, M.; Belden, B.; Hellerstein, S. & Alan, U. (1990). Nutritional and behavioural aspects of nasogastric tubefeeding in infants receiving chronic peritoneal dialysis. *Adv Perit Dial* 6:256-268

Zanakhshary, M.; Jamal, M.; Blair, GK.; Murphy, JJ.; Webber, EM. & Skarsgard, ED. (2005). Laparoscopic versus percutaneous endoscopic gastrostomy tube insertion: A new pediatric gold standard? *J Pediatr Surg.* 40:859-862

8

The Twin-Stoma Gastrostomy and the LOOPPEG® 3G Tube

Ah San, Pang
c/o Mount Alvernia Hospital
Singapore

1. Introduction

For tube feeding, the nasogastric tube and the percutaneous endoscopic gastrostomy (PEG) have been the main options, putting aside their minor variations, for decades. The relative relationship between these two options is illustrated in Figure 1. And the clinical evidence is undeniable: the nasogastric tube is low-comfort and low-risk whereas the PEG is high-comfort and high-risk.

For long-term use, patients and caregivers want a high-comfort and low-risk option (✓).

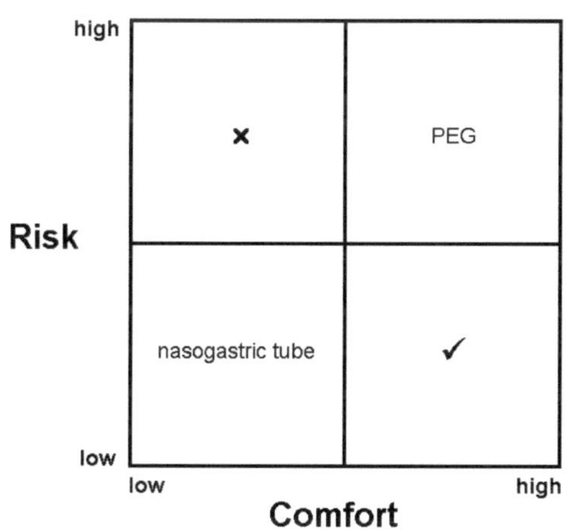

Fig. 1. The best-in-class option is high-comfort and low-risk

2. Why the nasogastric tube is low-comfort

The popular reason is the sensitive mucosal lining of the nose. Less often cited is the episodic increase in the effort of breathing caused by the tube. During upper respiratory tract infections, e.g. rhinorrhoea and rhinitis, the nasal mucosa becomes congested and oedematous. At these times, breathing through both nostrils is exhausting even for a normal person. For the patient with one nostril plugged by the tube and the other by mucus, the sensation is akin to suffocation.

Despite the use of soft materials like silicone, the nasogastric tube remains an uncomfortable option. A thinner tube will cause less discomfort but will choke faster. Tube exchange is far more distressing than a tube *in-situ*. Thus, from the comfort perspective, a thinner tube may not be a better deal because it must be exchanged more frequently.

The fault, if a normal structure can be faulted, lies with the nose and pharynx. Sneezing and gagging are basic reflexes. In a person who is unrestrained, if these reflexes do not clear the noxious stimulus (the tube), his hands and head will move to do so.

Clearly, to be a high-comfort option, the tube must bypass the nose and pharynx.

3. Why the PEG is high-risk

After more than 3 decades of clinical use, the complications associated with the PEG are well known (Gauderer, 2001).

The following complications have occurred because the PEG moved out of position: death, peritonitis, buried bumper syndrome, hemorrhage, oesophageal dislocation, intestinal obstruction, necrotizing fasciitis, track stenosis and loss of stoma. The following complications have occurred because of difficult tube exchange: track disruption, hemorrhage, peritonitis and death.

For the PEG, good tube security and easy tube exchange appear to be incompatible bedfellows. If the tube is anchored securely, it won't be easy to exchange. If made easy to exchange, it is not secure. Clearly, to be a low-risk option, the tube must always stay in position *and* must be easy to exchange.

4. Why the LOOPPEG® 3G tube is high-comfort and low-risk

The LOOPPEG® 3G tube, being a gastrostomy tube, is high-comfort because it by-passes the sensitive nose and pharynx. It is low-risk because it is devoid of complications which plaque the PEG.

It is a hollow silicone tube with the exit opening at its midpoint. Distances from the opening are marked on the tube. Each end is fitted with a dilator for pull-through like a PEG (Figure 2). After pull-through, the ends are crossed and locked together. When locked in this configuration, the tube cannot be dislodged, inward or outward. All the complications due to tube insecurity that plagued the PEG cannot happen.

The tube can be exchanged in four simple steps (Figure 3). First, unlock the old tube. Second, attach a new tube to any end of the old tube using the connector. Third, pull the other end of the old tube, removing it and guiding the new tube into position. Fourth, detach the old tube and lock the new tube. From a caregiver's perspective, it is easier to exchange the 3G tube than the nasogastric tube. All the complications due to difficult tube exchange that plagued the PEG cannot happen.

Visit www.looppeg.com for more information about this tube, the best in class. In the subsequent paragraphs, we will refer to it simply as the 3G tube. Other suitable names would be the loop-gastrostomy tube, u-tube, sg-tube, loop-PEG, buddy-PEG, twin-PEG and U-PEG.

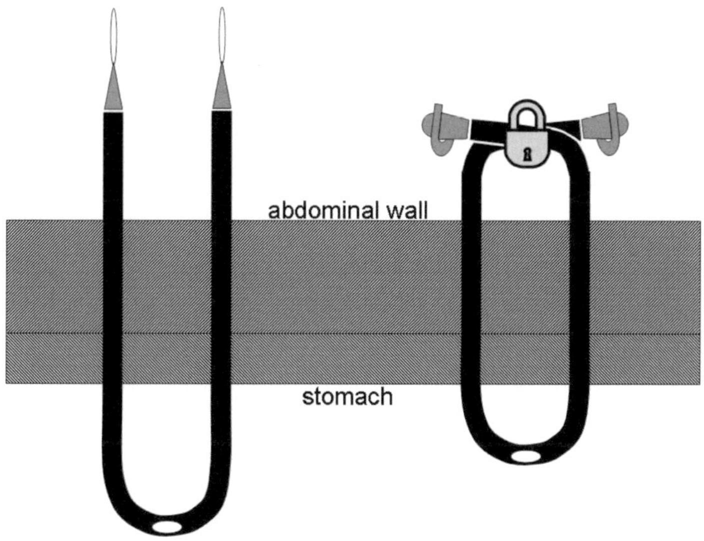

Fig. 2. LOOPPEG® 3G Tube

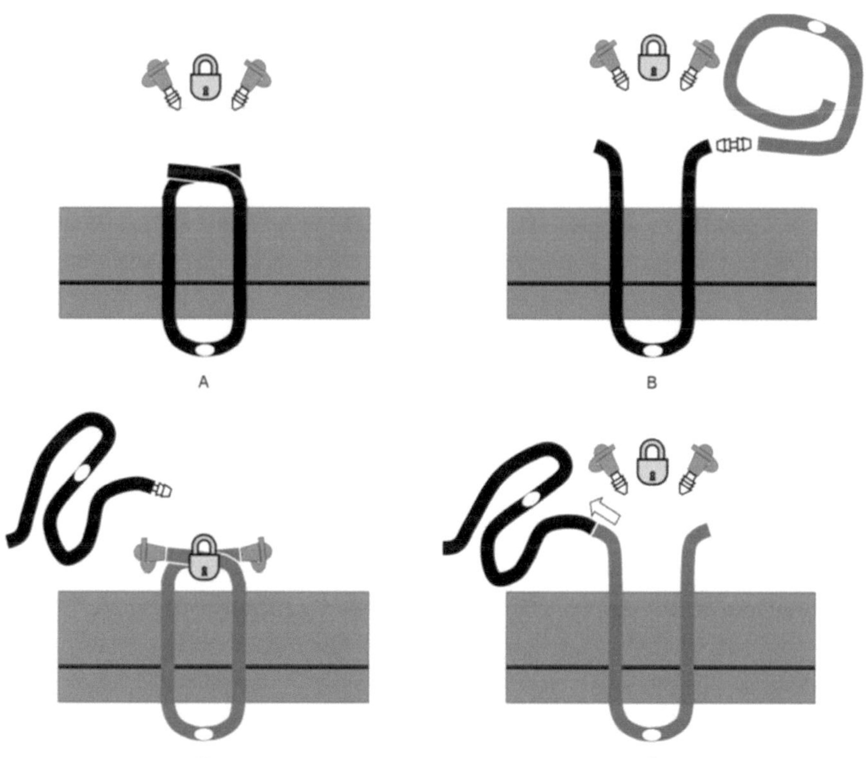

Fig. 3. LOOPPEG® 3G tube exchange is simple and easy

5. Portal *versus* Tube

We "blame" the sensitive mucosal lining for making the nasogastric tube low-comfort. Likewise, we blame the single stoma for the PEG being high-risk. Conversely, we credit the twin-stoma gastrostomy for making the 3G tube a high-comfort low-risk option.

It is easy to prove that portal is more important than tube. Take the 3G tube and use it with the other two portals. It will become low-comfort with one, and high-risk with the other. Then take other tubes and modify them for use with the twin-stoma gastrostomy; all will become high-comfort and low-risk. The inevitable conclusion is that the high-comfort low-risk profile is organic to the twin-stoma portal, not the tube.

To paraphrase Mark Twain, portal maketh the tube.

6. Why the twin-stoma gastrostomy is more effective

The term "twin-stoma gastrostomy" may be new but the concept, twinning for a better outcome, is not. Table 1 lists diverse examples where the concept has been successfully employed for a quantum improvement in performance.

The twin-stoma allows the use of a simple tube in a loop configuration, obviating the need for a balloon- or mushroom-shaped internal retaining structure. The single lock which keeps the tube in a loop configuration rests on normal skin, unlike the flange or bolster of the PEG. One end can be reserved for liquid food, and the other, liquid medicines.

The twin-stoma gastrostomy is akin to the dual PEG, used to treat gastric volvulus for the past 25 years (Altenwerth, 1994; Eckhauser & Ferron, 1985). Thus, it is a tried and tested procedure.

Singleton	**Twins**
Unicycle	Bicycle
Monohull boat	Catamaran
Single-engine aircraft	Twin-engine aircraft
Single-bolt lock	Double-bolt lock
One-key encryption	Two-key encryption
Single-point anchor	Two-point anchor
One-layer intestinal anastomosis	Two-layer intestinal anastomosis
Author	Co-authors

Table 1. Twinning is an established concept

7. Why the twin-stoma gastrostomy is safer

Suppose a large tube is split into halves, and the halves are converted into two smaller tubes. Since the total circumference of the two smaller tubes equals that of the large tube, the wounds are equal. Therefore, the twin-stoma is as large (safe) as the single-stoma, at worst.

There are two reasons why the twin-stoma may have a lower infection rate than the single stoma of equivalent size. First, a smaller sized tube has been shown to have a lower infection rate (Zopf *et al.*, 2008). Since the twin-stoma uses a small sized tube, the infection rate can be lower.

Second, a dirty tube predisposes to wound infection. We know that the PEG is so difficult to exchange that it is hardly exchanged at all, unless forced to by tube dysfunction (Sartori *et al.*, 2003). Thus, the PEG is prone to infection. In contrast, the 3G tube is very easy to exchange, and the caregiver can exchange it monthly or even fortnightly. Therefore, with more frequent tube exchanges, and better tube hygiene, the twin-stoma can have a lower infection rate.

Many medical examples of twinning to improve safety exist. A two-layer intestinal anastomosis has twice as many punctures as the single-layer anastomosis, each puncture created by the same needle. Yet it is accepted as safer by many surgeons. Another example is *double*-ligature of a major artery to keep hemorrhage at bay, practised by almost all surgeons. Most medical journals have a *two*-peer review process.

Thus, whether by way of analysis or medical example, the twin-stoma is safer than the single stoma.

8. How to add a gastropexy

Gastrostomy and gastropexy are related but separate moieties. By excluding the peritoneal cavity, the latter enhances the safety of the former.

For the twin-stoma gastrostomy, the gastropexy may be effected with T-fasteners or suturing. An alternative method is the loop-lock technique. A secondary loop is created at the midportion of the 3G tube with absorbable ligatures. Two ligatures, each comprising two square knots, are required (Figure 4). This is done before pull-through.

After pull-through, the secondary loop and lock are used to appose the stomach wall to the abdominal wall (Figure 5B). When the LOOPPEG® is used in this fashion, we refer to it as the LOOPPEGG™ (the additional G to represent the gastropexy).

A polyglactin 3/0 ligature will undergo gastric acid hydrolysis and release the secondary loop about 30 days later (Chu, 1982). This duration is sufficient for adhesions to develop. If a longer duration is desired, polydioxanone may be selected (Hoile, 1983). Release is easily detected; the lock is lifted off the skin (Figure 5D).

Our current practice is to always insert the 3G tube with a secondary loop. Besides providing traction, the secondary loop keeps the central opening of the tube within the stomach and away from the gastric puncture sites.

Tube exchange using the percutaneous method (Figure 3) cannot be done unless the secondary loop is released. Thus, do not select a ligature material which takes a long time to biodegrade. Ideally, the material should biodegrade after adhesions have formed but before tube exchange is due. If tube exchange (or removal) is required before release, it must be done endoscopically.

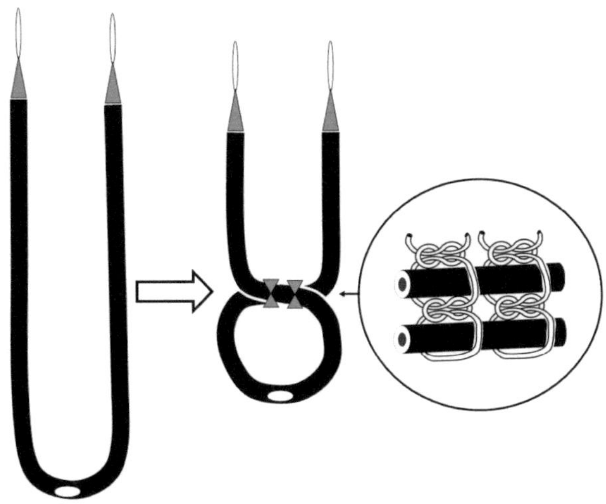

Fig. 4. The secondary loop is created with absorbable ligatures

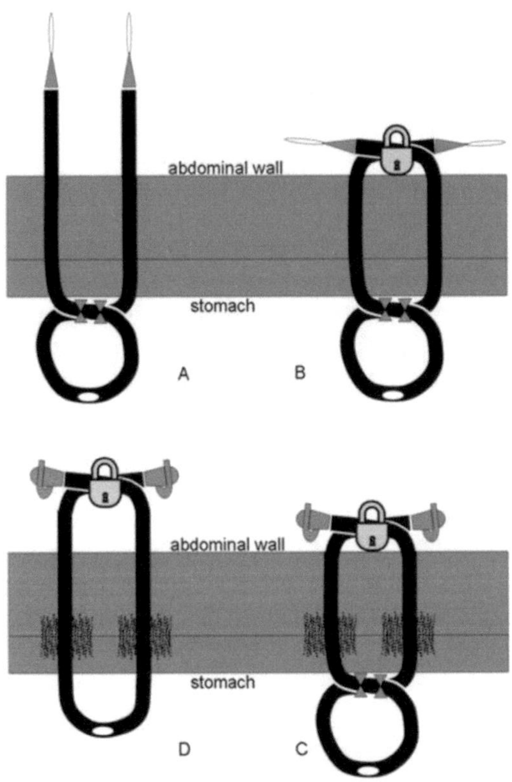

Fig. 5. The secondary loop is created before pull-through (A). The secondary loop and lock keep stomach apposed to abdominal wall (B). Adhesions develop with time (C). The lock is lifted off the skin when the ligatures undergo biodegradation, and release the secondary loop (D)

9. How to convert the single-stoma PEG to twin-stoma gastrostomy

Where feasible, the stoma occupied by the PEG should be used as one of the twin stomas. In this way, a matured track is not wasted; only one extra gastric puncture is needed.

If there is a size discrepancy, the PEG stoma is likely to be too loose for the 15 Fr 3G tube. Parenteral feeding may be used while the track stenose spontaneously to provide a snug fit.

For removal of the PEG, we recommend the technique described by Turner *et al.* (2010). The technique involves transfixion-ligature of the PEG. It is helpful to keep the end of the transfixion-ligature long for easy retrieval by a tripod snare. Removal is done after initial gastroscopy and the extra gastric puncture. If this sequence is not followed, air leak from the PEG stoma may cause loss of gastric distension, and interfere with the conduct of the conversion.

10. The road ahead

The twin-stoma gastrostomy and the 3G tube refer to the same thing, the best-in-class option (Figure 1). They are suitable for extended-term use; for patients who tend to pull on their tubes (e.g. mental retardation and dementia); for situations demanding stringent hygiene and frequent tube exchange (e.g. diabetes mellitus); and for places where access to medical facilities is limited (e.g. physically vast country).

22% of physically restrained residents in nursing homes in Singapore were "abused" to protect their nasogastric tubes from being pulled out (Mamun & Lim, 2005). In the Netherlands, a developed country, 22% of patients with nasogastric tubes were physically restrained for the same reason (Baeten & Hoefnagels, 1992). We hope the twin-stoma gastrostomy will encourage caregivers to convert their patients, reduce misuse of the nasogastric tube, and nip needless immobilisation by physical restraints.

A few doctors disagree with the use of the PEG in the demented elderly (Akner, 2005). What tipped the balance might have been its high-risk relative to the few months of remaining life. If so, the availability of the low-risk 3G tube should invite a re-think. The lack of improved survival with a feeding tube should not be a reason to reject it. After all, Medicine is not just about cure. More often, it is about caring and compassion, making the journey "less inhumane" for a loved one who will depart soon. The feeding tube can provide palliative decompression too (Pang, 2011).

Others believe that the gastrostomy tube should be established early, not late (Figueiredo *et al.*, 2007). For them, the twin-stoma gastrostomy (or 3G tube) should help their cause.

11. Misconceptions

At the roadshows of the 3G tube for doctors, a frequent question posed to us was whether it had been "proven to be safe and effective with a randomized controlled trial (RCT)." This misconception immediately tells two things about the questioner. First, he is not a general surgeon. The practicing general surgeon, or one capable of anything more complex than a gastrectomy, from operative experience, knows intuitively that the 3G tube is safe and effective.

Second, the questioner is not conversant with the limitations of a RCT. Randomization is just a means to control bias in a study, in this case an experiment in human beings. After randomization, if the test group is given the 3G tube, the control group would not be given it. In other words, the control group will get a sham tube. Two issues become apparent. Isn't the study, particularly the control (sham tube) arm, unethical? Isn't the conclusion, specifically the finding in the test group, predicable? Of course, the answer is yes for both. Thus, the bona fide general surgeon will not conduct a RCT on the 3G tube, for no reason other than he is ethical and does not perform sham operations. (This is not to say that he cannot collect a case series, and report it in a medical journal. My own cases have been reported elsewhere.)

Another misconception is that the 3G tube should not be allowed into mainstream practice unless it has been shown to prolong patient survival. But a feeding tube cannot cure the dysphagic patient of his primary condition, be it stroke, dementia, Parkinsonism, cancer, motor neurone disease, etc. Many of these patients will die soon after they become dependent on the feeding tube. It is unreasonable to expect the 3G tube to be a miracle drug.

The 3G tube is a device, not a drug. Its effects are "local and predictable" in the words of the Food and Drug Administration of the United States of America. It is silly to obstruct its introduction into clinical practice, or deny the patient his rights to have a secure and easy to exchange gastrostomy tube, using oppressive and irrelevant requirements like "Phase I – IV clinical trials".

Yet another common misconception is that two stomas will cause more pain to the patient. While this is true if we use a 3G tube which is as large as the PEG, it need not be so. A fine bore tube can always be used as the 3G tube because we are not bothered by tube blockage. If blockage happens, we can simply and easily exchange the tube. In contrast, we always need to use the largest PEG tolerable by the patient. With the PEG, we dread blockage; we want to avoid having to exchange a blocked PEG and all the attendant dangers.

Critics of the 3G tube tend to harp: "The insertion of the loop PEG requires more steps than the PEG. Why should I do the more difficult operation?" These critics have forgotten the Hippocratic Oath. PEG tube dislodgements are extremely traumatic events: physically, psychologically and financially, for the victim, not the doctor (Pang & Low). Doing a simpler PEG operation may result in a lifetime of worry about tube accidents for the patient and his family. On the other hand, the 3G tube, more "difficult" for the doctor - by virtue of one more gastric puncture with a 14G needle - will lessen the burden of care for the patient. To turn away from the 3G tube is to turn a blind eye to the plight of dysphagic patients (Pang & Maetani, 2011).

Early adopters of the 3G tube should be aware of a bizarre hazard. Until the rationale of the twin-stoma becomes widely known, it will appear that these adopters have violated their patients with an unnecessary extra wound. They may find themselves hauled by their rivals to appear before the regulatory authority to answer a charge of professional misconduct. Strange as it may seem here, it did happen to me.

12. Conclusion

The twin-stoma gastrostomy, high-comfort and low-risk, is the option for all seasons. One complete approach is provided by the LOOPPEG® 3G tube. For the cost of a strand of absorbable material, a gastropexy can be added.

13. Acknowledgements

The Franciscan Missionaries of the Divine Motherhood in Singapore provided the author with opportunity, space and inspiration, without which the 3G tube would not have been invented. For the record, the FMDM nuns did not agree to be acknowledged. But their selflessness was all the more worthy of acknowledging. SGN Pte Ltd (www.looppeg.com) funded the Article Processing Charge. To Dr Chia Siew Cheng, this article is dedicated.

14. References

Akner G. (2005). PEG treatment: an increasing dilemma. *Age and Ageing*, Vol.34, No.4, pp. 320-321, ISSN 0002-0729

Altenwerth FJ. (1994). [Treatment of an intermittent stomach volvulus using gastropexy via percutaneous endoscopic gastrostomy]. *Deutsche medizinische Wochenschrift*, Vol.110, No.48, pp. 1658-1660, ISSN 0012-0472

Baeten C & Hoefnagels J. (1992). Feeding via nasogastric tube or percutaneous endoscopic gastrostomy. A comparison. *Scandinavian Journal of Gastroenterology*, Vol.27, No.s194, pp. 95-98, ISSN 0036-5521

Chu CC. (1982). A comparison of the effect of pH on the biodegradation of two synthetic absorbable sutures. *Annals of Surgery*, Vol.195, No.1, pp.55-59, ISSN 0003-4932

Eckhauser ML & Ferron JP. (1985). The use of dual percutaneous endoscopic gastrostomy (DPEG) in the management of chronic intermittent gastric volvulus. *Gastrointestinal Endoscopy*, Vol.31 No.5, pp. 340-342, ISSN 0016-5107

Figueiredo FA, da Costa MC, Pelosi AD, Martins RN, Machado L & Francioni E. (2007). Predicting outcomes and complications of percutaneous endoscopic gastrostomy. *Endoscopy*, Vol.39, No.4, pp. 333-338, ISSN 1438-8812

Gauderer MW. (2001). Percutaneous endoscopic gastrostomy - 20 years later: a historical perspective. *Journal of Pediatric Surgery*, Vol.36, No.1, pp. 217-219, ISSN 0022-3468

Hoile RW. (1983). The use of a new suture material (Polydioxanone) in the biliary tract. *Annals of the Royal College of Surgeons of England*, Vol.65, No.3, pp. 168-171, ISSN 0035-8843

Mamun K & Lim J. (2005). Use of physical restraints in nursing homes: current practice in Singapore. *Annals of the Academy of Medicine, Singapore*, Vol.34, No.2, pp. 158-162, ISSN 0304-4602

Pang AS. (2011). A Feeding Tube Can Be Used for Palliative Decompression Too. *Journal of Palliative Medicine*, Vol.14, No.4, pp. 388, ISSN 1096-6218

Pang AS & Maetani I. (2011). The Road Ahead for Percutaneous Endoscopic Gastrostomy - Defiance or Deliverance. *Internal Medicine*, Vol. 50, No. 8, pp. 949, ISSN 0918-2918

Pang AS & Low JM. (2011). Twin-stoma gastrostomy. *ANZ Journal of Surgery*, Vol. 81, No. 7-8, pp. 575-576, ISSN 1445-2197

Sartori S, Trevisani L, Nielsen I, Tassinari D, Ceccotti P & Abbasciano V. (2003). Longevity of silicone and polyurethane catheters in long-term enteral feeding via percutaneous endoscopic gastrostomy. *Alimentary Pharmacology & Therapeutics*, Vol.17, No.6, pp. 853-856, ISSN 0269-2813

Turner JK, Berrill JW, Dolwani S, Green JT & Swift G. (2010). Percutaneous endoscopic gastrostomy tube placement. *Endoscopy*, Vol.42, No.S02, pp.E146-E147, ISSN 1438-8812

Zopf Y, Konturek P, Nuernberger A, Maiss J, Zenk J, Iro H, Hahn EG & Schwab D. (2008). Local infection after placement of percutaneous endoscopic gastrostomy tubes: A prospective study evaluating risk factors. *Canadian Journal of Gastroenterology*, Vol. 22, No. 12, pp. 987-991, ISSN 0835-7900

Part 4

Complications of Gastrostomy

9

High Level of Intra-Gastric Pressure is Risk Factor for Patients with Percutaneous Endoscopic Gastrostomy (PEG)

Michiaki Kudo, Nobuyuki Kanai, Toshiaki Hirasawa,
Takayuki Asao and Hiroyuki Kuwano
*Department of General Surgical Science (Surgery I),
Gunma University, Graduate School of Medicine
Japan*

1. Introduction

In Japan, percutaneous endoscopic gastrostomy (PEG) has been used mainly in patients with stroke and dementia, who are unable to undertake oral ingestion voluntarily. The number of patients who rely on PEG feeding has recently increasing. The occurrence of aspiration pneumonia after PEG placement is difficult to predict. With a simple and new examination procedure which measures intra-gastric pressure (IGP) during the hungry period, we were able to determine the presence of aspiration pneumonia in PEG patients. Sixty patients living in a home-care type facility or nursing home were examined in our hospital from November, 2010 to January 2011. The patient lies down horizontally in the supine position. IGP is measured using a PEG tube. Using like this method, the intra-abdominal pressure (IAP) is measured in cases of the abdominal compartment syndrome, while central venous pressure (CVP) is measured in cases of heart disorder. The mean IGP in patients without complicated pneumonia was 2.1 ± 1.7 cmH_2O. In patients with complicated pneumonia ($p<0.0001$), it was 7.9 ± 2.7 cm H_2O. There is a relationship between IGP and the symptoms of aspiration pneumonia. Our simple and easy technique can estimate the level of complication and can assist in the prevention of pneumonia in patients living in nursing facilities.

2. Prognostic significance of intra-gastric pressure for the occurrence of aspiration pneumonia

Percutaneous endoscopic gastrosotomy (PEG) tubes have been used mainly in the patients with stroke and dementia who are unable to undertake oral ingestion voluntary. PEG feeding nutrition has been reported to be an effective and safe procedure with a low incidence of complications. Nevertheless, with increased use by many patients in serious condition and among very old patients, complications have been encountered more frequently in recent years in Japan. One of the most common complications is aspiration pneumonia and PEG tube problems such as obstruction accompanied with pollution inside the tube. There have been several reports of cases of PEG patients having died as a result of aspiration pneumonia (1, 2).

Due to the benefits of enteral nutrition and with improvements in PEG patient management, the number of PEG patients has increased remarkably. However, the placement and management of PEG tubes are not without risks (3, 4). The overall complication rate has remained stable over the last 15-20 years, ranging from 4 % to 23.8 % of cases. Three to 4% of all cases are affected by major complications, i.e. those that are life threatening and/or require surgical intervention or hospitalization. More common minor complications occur in between 7.4% and 20.0% of cases (5).

In many cases, PEG patients live in home-care facilities or nursing homes which lack the more sophisticated instruments available in hospitals. It is necessary to distinguish patients for whom complications can easily arise from patients for whom complications are unlikely. Our new technique measures intra-gastric pressure (IGP) for the purpose of screening for high risk cases of aspiration pneumonia (6). This examination technique is a modification of that technique being used to measure intra-abdominal pressure (IAP) in the case of the abdominal compartment syndrome (7) and for measuring central venous pressure (CVP) to monitor cardiac function and so on (8). A rise of IGP causes the reflux to the esophagus from the stomach. And as a result of aspiration of gastric juice to the lung, symptoms of aspiration pneumonia occur. We can prevent aspiration pneumonia by monitoring IGP.

We have confirmed that a relationship between pneumonia and a high IGP level exists, and hope to introduce this safe, simple and effective bedside technique for evaluating patients living in home-care facilities, in the hope that we can decrease complications such as the pneumonia and the obstruction of the PEG tube.

2.1 Materials and methods

Sixty consecutive patients (23 men, aged 49-89 and 37 women, aged 43-90) who had received a medical examination with PEG catheter, were studied from November 2010 to January 2011. A PEG tube of from 20 to 24 Fr in diameter had been inserted as the primary means of long-term nutrition in patients with swallowing disorders. It had been 3 months since the PEG operation. In many cases, patients had been maintained in home-care type facilities or nursing homes lacking hospital-level medical instruments.

The patient lies down horizontally in the supine position. Intra-gastric pressure is measured directly using the PEG catheter over 6-8 respiratory cycles in the empty period. First, the air in the stomach is aspirated, and we put into 50 ml of warm water in the syringe into the PEG tube and the stomach. We measure the height from the top of the skin of the abdomen to the surface of the water in the PEG tube (Fig. 1). We wait several minutes and measure when the IGP value is high. The height of the surface of the water is unstable; however, the value can be measured at the center. We repeat the same technique three times and we average the results

Patients were classified into two groups. In the first group there was no suspicion of pneumonia while in the second group pneumonia was complicated. The first group contained of 19 men aged 44-89 and 30 women aged 46-89. The second group consisted of four men aged 48-86 and 7 women aged 43-90. For all cases, diatrizoate (Gastrografin) study was performed. Gastrografin 30 ml was given by using PEG tube, and confirmed that the PEG tube was in proper position in the stomach and the discharge from the stomach to the duodenum was normal. Finally, the gastro-esophageal reflux and the movement and function of the stomach are confirmed carefully.

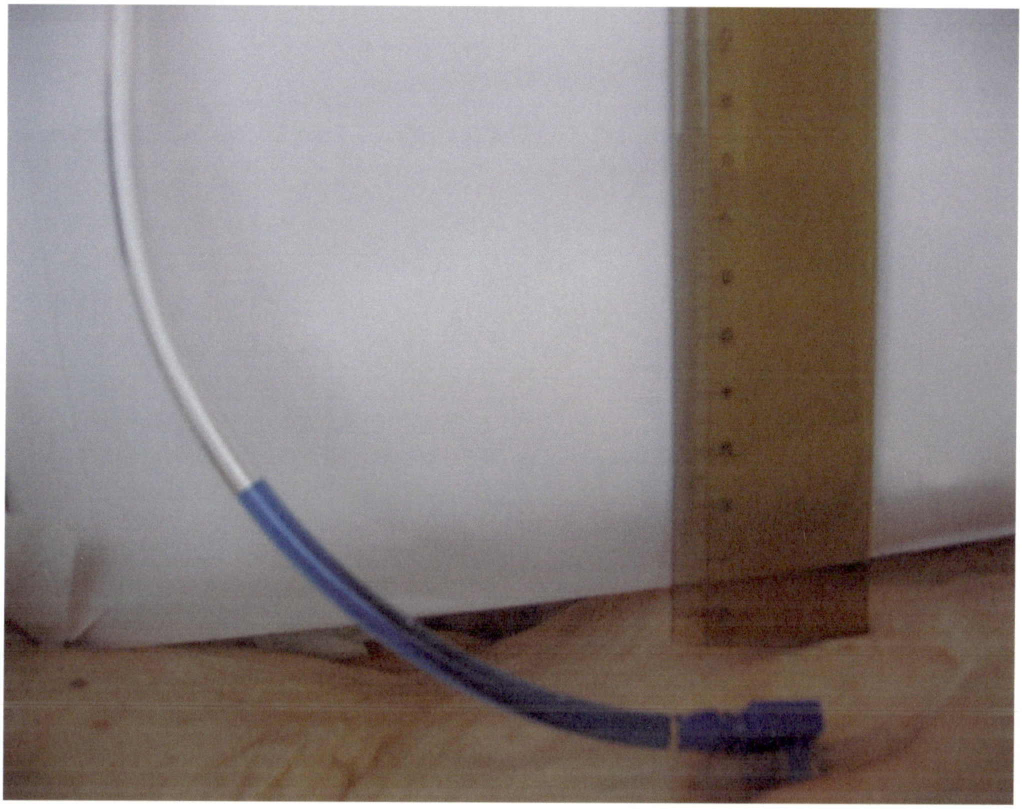

Fig. 1. The technique of measuring intra-gastric pressure using PEG tube. The patient lies down horizontally in the supine position. The water contains 0.1 mg/ml Indigocarmine. Intra-gastric pressures show 3 cmH_2O in this case

A chest x-ray, a body temperature over 37.5 degrees C, pulse rate is over 100 beats/min and listening to the lungs with a stethoscope (auscultation), were criteria used to diagnose pneumonia.

2.2 Statistical analysis

The data was stored on Microsoft Excel Office 2007 and processed using SPSS Scientific package SPSS 12.0 (SPSS Inc., Chicago, IL). Statistical significance of the changes in routines was evaluated by χ^2 and Fisher exact test. Results were considered to be statistically significant at an alpha of 0.05.

2.3 Results of intra-gastric pressure of PEG patient

The median IGP was 2.1 ± 1.7 cmH_2O for patients who were not suffering from complicated pneumonia (n=49) and 7.9 ± 2.7 cmH_2O for patients who were suffering from complicated pneumonia (n=11) ($p < 0.0001$)(Fig. 2). In cases where the pneumonia was not complicated, IGP was lower than 8 cm. The rate of IGP was equal to or greater than 7 cm was 0%. While in cases involving complicated pneumonia and the rate of IGP was equal to or greater than 7 cm, it was 63.6%.

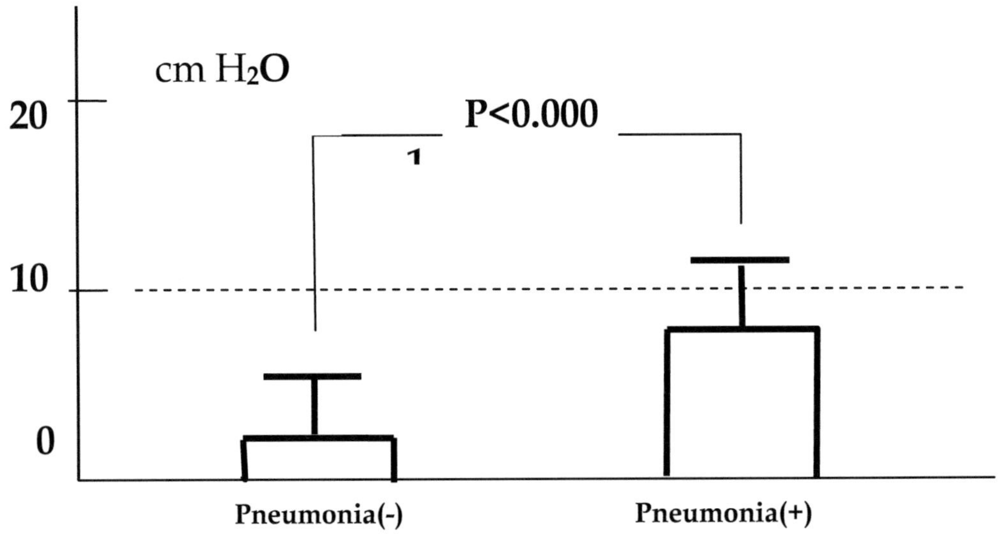

Fig. 2. Intra-gastric pressure (IGP) cm H_2O

Intra-gastric pressure of PEG patient. The median IGP were 2.1 ± 1.7 cmH_2O for the patient without complicated pneumonia and 7.9 ± 2.7 cmH_2O for the patient with complicated pneumonia ($p < 0.0001$).

2.4 Discussion

Percutaneous endoscopic gastrostomy (PEG) is generally used for long-term enteral nutrition in patients with prolonged swallowing difficulties and inabilities. Patients requiring PEG placement are often very sick, and suffer from postoperative complications. One such complication, aspiration pneumonia, can be especially fatal. Complications encountered in a large series of studies have demonstrated that procedure-related mortality occurred in less than 1%, of major complications and in 3% of minor complications in less than 14% of patients(9). During observation after PEG operation, the occurrence of aspiration pneumonia is well recognized. Over 70 % of causes of death after PEG operation at our hospital were aspiration pneumonia even if the gastrografin study is normal in the stable postoperative condition (6). Therefore, an examination aimed at prevention of pneumonia in PEG patients is needed.

Moreover, physicians who place PEG tubes endoscopically often do not have the opportunity to provide these patients with long-term follow up care (10). Thus, those nutrition support specialists who do treat PEG patients may be different than those members of the health care team who are in the most advantageous position for ongoing inspection and maintenance of the access devices. Dietitians, wound-care ostomy nurses, and other nutrition support specialists are encouraged to be more proactive with their participation in the care and management of the PEG site. However, because all the members are not experts in PEG, simple methods for identifying problems are necessary.

In preventing complications in PEG patients, inspection techniques are of primary importance.

When a patient develops a distended and taunt abdomen in the case of the abdominal injury, the measurement of abdominal compartment pressure can help with early recognition of organ dysfunction (7). Normal IGP is 0-5 mmHg (0-7 cmH_2O). At 10 mmHg, the cardiac output may begin to decrease. Hypotension and oliguria can occur at 15 to 20 mmHg (20-26 cmH_2O), and anuria will occur with pressure over 40 mmHg. The collective effects of the increased abdominal pressure are called Abdominal Compartment Syndrome. When pressure in the abdominal compartment overcomes the pressure inside the capillaries perfusing the organs of the abdomen, ischemia and infarction of the organ can occur.

The reason for measuring intra-abdominal pressure is due to the following structure (7). The bladder is an extraperitoneal, intra-abdominal structure with a very soft wall. Because of this, changes in intra-abdominal pressure are reflected in changes in bladder pressure. When the bladder is filled with 50 to 100 ml of fluid, there is virtually no pressure exerted on the bladder wall, allowing it to act as a passive pressure monitor. A foley catheter can be then used to monitor for abdominal compartment syndrome. Failure to recognize and treat intra-abdominal hypertension will results in increased risk of renal impairment, visceral and intestinal ischemia, respiratory failure and death.

From a similar point of view, CVP is clinically applied to monitor cardiac function. CVP is an indicator of cardiac preload and reflects right ventricular function (8). In most cases, left heart function correlates well with right heart function. Considering the above, measuring IGP by using the PEG tube was useful for determination of the patient's condition.

IGP has also been used for other purposes. For example, IGP is used to estimate abdominal wall hernia formation following surgery. The mean pressures of males and females do not differ. And, it has been reported that the mean IAP for sitting and standing is 16.7 and 20 mm Hg respectively. Coughing and jumping generate the highest IAP (107.6 and 171 mmHg, respectively) (11).

The endoscopist who places PEG tubes is not often concerned with long-term management and follow-up care in PEG patients. There needs to be a system for identifying complications more easily. It is important that the measurement of IGP in PEG patients can be determined easily without any special instrument.

According to our measurements, the median IGP of patients with complicated pneumonia were 7.9 ± 2.7 cmH_2O, and 2.1 ± 1.7 cmH_2O and for patients without complicated pneumonia ($p < 0.0001$). We reported the similar results in the previous manuscript in 2008(6) and confirmed that by the results of our measurement, the median IGP of the patient who complicated pneumonia were 10.4 ± 7.1 cmH_2O, and 4.7 ± 4.5 cmH_2O for the patient who did not have complicated pneumonia ($p < 0.0001$). The higher pressure reflects the status of the pneumonia. Based on our observations, patients who have symptoms of pneumonia appear to generate a significant elevation in IGP, and IGP reflects the prognosis of PEG patients by a similar method of IAP and CVP. In cases of complicated pneumonia, the rate of IGP over 7 cmH_2O was 63.6 %.On the other hand, in cases without complicated pneumonia, the rate of IGP over 7 cmH_2O was 0%. Cases in which IGP is equal to or greater than 7 cm H_2O, may possibly be complicated pneumonia.

The highest intra-abdominal pressure in healthy patients is generated during coughing. And, coughing is a symptom of pneumonia. Therefore, the IGP of patients with pneumonia increases. The measurement of IGP is also related to physiological conditions.

Among elderly people such as PEG patients, the lower esophageal sphincter (LES) pressure shows a greater decrease than in younger people (12, 13). Consequently, for elderly people, the risk of aspiration pneumonia is higher than it is in younger people. We confirmed gastro-esophageal reflux by the Gastrografin study. The result showed that the reflex is recognized in only thirteen of one hundred thirty -two cases (9.8%) (6). we need further examination to determinate the condition of PEG patients from these results (date not shown) (14).

Serious complications related PEG tubes which can not be predicted were reported several months after PEG placement. For example, a case of prolonged duodenal paralysis after PEG replacement in a patient with traumatic brain injury was reported in 2011 (15). This case report describes an uncommon complication of PEG placement in a vegetative state after traumatic brain injury: the development of prolonged duodenal paralysis. This patient was treated by placement of a transient jejunostomy until recovery of duodenal function activity, to permit adequate nutrition. This transient jejunostomy for duodenal paralysis has been previously unreported. In this case, persistent high level of IGP is expected, the aggravation of the symptom can be prevented.

Buried bumper syndrome is a serious complication related to PEG tubes and needs hospital treatment (16). It is difficult to diagnose from the appearance of the PEG tube and vital signs of the patient. Computed tomography examination of the abdomen is effective to reveal buried bumper syndrome. But in many cases, patients live in a nursing facilities or at home. In addition, buried bumper syndrome is not uncommon and can occur soon after insertion of a PEG tube. The buried tube can be safely removed by external traction and in most cases can then be replaced with a pull-type or balloon replacement tube by expert doctor (17). It is essential that the condition be easily recognized without any instrument at nursing facilities and in the patient's home. In cases of buried bumper syndrome, IGP is assumed to be approximately 0 cm H_2O. Although buried bumper syndrome is still relatively uncommon, it may be a complication that deserves increasing attention because PEG tube replacement is expected to be used more frequently in the future (18).

Incorrect insertion of the PEG tube that may occur in case of PEG tube replacement is a common complication. This changeover complication may seriously affect the patient's nutrition, so it is important to detect it early. The frequency of incorrect insertion of the balloon gastrostomy tube is lower than that of the bumper type PEG tube. Although the balloon gastrostomy tube may be used as alternative to PEG tubes in patients on long-term enterable feeding in the community, the higher cost of using balloon gastrostomy tube over PEG tubes should be considered when selecting feeding tubes for patients in community (19). In many cases of the patient utilize bumper type PEG tube feeding. Correct replacement of PEG tube can be confirmed by Gastrografin study or endoscopic examination at the hospital. It is possible to confirm this complication by comparing IGP before and after exchange PEG tube. If the staff at the nursing facilities or patient's family measure IGP, it is possible to suspect that some problem has occurred after PEG tube replacement.

PEG proved an effective method for enteral nutrition (20), and many people have been able to return to their home (21). The appropriate training of care professionals and familiar supporters in charge of the patients carrying a PEG tube ensures its continuous functioning and reduces the risk of complications (22). A system for identifying complication more easily is important, and the measurement of IGP in PEG patients can be determined easily without the need for any special instrument.

3. Conclusion

There is a relationship between IGP and the symptoms of aspiration pneumonia. Our simple and easy technique can estimate the level of complication and can assist in the prevention of pneumonia in patients living in nursing facilities and at home. We conclude that our technique is useful in monitoring PEG patients and in preventing aspiration pneumonia and other complications related to PEG feeding. Indeed, it is not possible to prevent aspiration pneumonia in all cases, but higher IGP is one of the causes of aspiration pneumonia. We believe that this technique will prove to be an effective technique for monitoring PEG patients under a network of integrated services.

4. Acknowledgment

We wish to thank Dr. Nobuo Takahashi for valuable cooperation and excellent technical assistance. And we wish to thank Prof. Allen Meyer for special advice about description.

5. References

[1] Callahan CM, Haag KM, Weinberger M, Tierney WM, Buchanan NN, Stump TE, Nishi R. Outcomes of percutaneous endoscopic gastrostomy among adults in a community setting. J Am Geriatr Soc, 2000; 48:1048-54
[2] Grant MD, Rudberg MA, Brody JA. Gastrostomy placement and mortality among hospitalized Medicare beneficiaries. JAMA, 1998; 279: 1973-6
[3] Larson DE, Burton DD, Schroeder KW, DiMagno EP. Percutaneous endoscopic gastrostomy. Indications, success, complications, and mortality in 314 consecutive patients. Gastroenterology, 1987; 93: 48-52.
[4] Rabeneck L, Wray NP, Petersen NJ. Long-term outcomes of patients receiving percutaneous endoscopic gastrostomy tubes. J Gen Intern Med, 1996; 11: 287-293
[5] Loser C, Wolters S, Folsch UR. Enteral long-term nutrition via percutaneous endoscopic gastrosotomy (PEG) in 210 patients: a four-year prospective study. Dig Dis Sci, 1998; 43: 2549-57
[6] Kudo M, Kanai N, Hirasawa T, Asao T, Kuwano H. Prognostic significance of intragastric pressure for the occurrence of aspiration pneumonia in the patients with percutaneous endoscopic gastrostomy (PEG). Hepatogastroenterolpgy 2008; 55: 1935-8
[7] Sugrue M. Abdominal compartment syndrome. Curr Opin Crit Care. 2005; 11(4): 333-8
[8] Magder S, Bafaqeeh F. The clinical role of central venous pressure measurement. J Intensive Care Med. 2007; 22: 44-51
[9] Chen W, Kawahara H, Takahashi M, Matsushima A, Takase S. Marked pneumoperitoneum 3 weeks after percutaneous endoscopic gastrostomy. J Gastroenterol Hepatol. 2006; 21: 919-921
[10] McClave SA, Neff RL. Care and long-term maintenance of percutaneous endoscopic gastrostomy tubes. J Parenter Enteral Nutr. 2006; 30(1 Suppl): S27-38
[11] Cobb WS, Burns JM, Kercher KW et al. Normal intraabdominal pressure in healthy adults. J Surg Res. 2005; 129: 231-5
[12] Mittal RK, McCallum RW. Characteristics of transient lower esophageal sphincter relaxation in humans. Am J Physiol 1987; 252(5 Pt 1): G636-41

[13] Dodds WJ, Dent J, Hogan WJ et al. Mechanism of gastroesophageal reflux in patients with reflux esophagitis. N Engl J Med. 1982; 307: 1547-521
[14] Attanasio A, Bedin M, Stocco S, Negrin V, Biancon A, Cecchetto G, Tagliapietra M. Clinical outcomes and complications of enteral nutrition among older adults. Minerva Med. 2009, 100: 159-66
[15] Mammi P, Zaccaria B, Dazzi F, Saccavini M. Prolonged duodenal paralysis after PEG placement in a patient with traumatic brain injury: a case report. Eur J Phys Rehabil Med. 2011; 47: 49-51
[16] Johnson T, Velez KA, Zhan E. Buried bumper syndrome causing rectus abdominis necrosis in a man with tetraplegia. Spinal Cord. 2010; 48: 85-6
[17] Lee TH, Lin JT. Clinical manifestations and management of buried bumper syndrome in patients with percutaneous endoscopic gastrostomy. Gastrointest Endosc. 2008; 68: 580-4
[18] Sasaki T, Fukumori D, Sano M, Sakai K, Ohmori H, Yamamoto F. Percutaneous endoscopic gastrostomy complicated by buried bumper syndrome. Int Surg. 2003; 88: 64-7
[19] Ojo. Balloon gastrostomy tubes for long-term feeding in the community. Br J Nurs. 2011; 20: 34-8
[20] Lempa M, Kohler L, Frusemers O. Troidl H. Percutaneous endoscopic gastrostomy (PEG). Course, nutrition and care in 233 consecutive patients. Fortschr Med Orig. 2002; 120: 143-6
[21] Abitbol V, Selinger-Leneman H, Gallais Y, Piette F, Bouchon JP, Piera JB, Beinis JY, Laurent M, Moulias R, Gaudric M. Percutaneous endoscopic gastrostomy in elderly patients. A prospective study in a geriatric hospital. Gastroenterol Clin Biol. 2002; 26: 488-53
[22] Friginal-Ruiz AB, Gonzalez-Castillo S, Lucendo AJ. Endoscopic percutaneous gastrostomy: an update on the indications, technique and nursing care. Enferm Clin. 2011; 21: 173-78

Part 5

Psychosomatic Aspects of Gastrostomy

10

Psychosomatic Manifestations of Gastrostomy in Head and Neck Surgery

Francisco Hernández Altemir[1,2], Sofía Hernández Montero[3,4,5], Susana Hernández Montero[6], Elena Hernández Montero[7] and Manuel Moros Peña[8]

[1]*University of Zaragoza,*
[2]*European Association for Cranio-Maxillofacial Surgery and the Head and Neck Surgery,*
[3]*Association and the New Head and Neck Spain Association*
[4]*University Master of Oral Implants and Prostodontic, UAX Madrid,*
[5]*Zaragoza University,*
[6]*Zaragoza University (Medicine Oral and Pathology) Endodontic,*
[7]*ORL Viladecans Hospital and Institute García Ibáñez of Otoneurosurgery, Barcelona*
[8]*Pediatric and Cartoonist*
Spain

1. Introduction

There are several pathologies that can demand the indication and practice of Gastrostomies in patients with pathologies in head and neck areas, from patients with diverse medical aetiology affection to others with pathologies that register in the surgical scope.

We are going to deal with, as the title indicates, those patients that essentially are derived from patients of the scope of surgery, although we will not totally leave the gastrostomies in patients with anatomical and /or functional affections located properly in the territory of oral and craniofacial or whose origin can be far from this, as the case of patients with more or less global and complex syndromes that repels in elementary function of a relationship. Like the ear, the language, the sight, and the oral structures and as in the case that occupies us, the feeding.

The recent incorporation of the face transplants has been able to awake in us a bigger feeling even more than it already did over the isolation and dependency that these patients suffer, besides all what a surgery of this spread entails, valuing the meaning that this can represent to them seeing themselves forced to support the loss of a habit so primitive and natural as it can be eating by ordinary routes, this is going to be on addition to what the transplanted patient is going to support such as isolation, being too long in bed, tracheotomy, tarsorrhaphy, more or less complex monitoring, drainages, droppers through central and peripheral vessels for very prolonged periods of time, urinary catheter, intermaxillary blocks, ... etc. that altogether, is going to decrease his independence, and he will have to depend on other persons and/ or machines, artifices and even robots, all this is going to decrease or reduce their freedom and capacities of expression and self- esteem. Their primitive liberties to move, to communicate and to be made understood, to eat by the

natural routes and to be able to chew, to swallow safely and to savor foods, also to move their hands and members in general, and all of this with a more or functionless face.
Further on, we will incorporate and develop a novel term or maybe two, that have lots to do with what we are explaining in this chapter, organintegration (O), and or better Pseudoorganintegration (PsO), that comes to synthesize in several psychopathological aspects, which first of all means for the patient as a receiver, his family and the society in general and specially for the professionals in medicine, understanding that we are in front of a special almost unique situation by the organization of the act and what it means to the above mentioned to understand in a clear way, the patients as a receiver of a compound tissue, as can be a face, faces multitude of unsuspicious circumstances, perceptions, and situations no matter how much preparation he had previously. We will denominate them in the text as (O) and or (PsO).

2. Psychosomatic manifestations

When we talk about the psychosomatic manifestations in gastrostomized patients, we must understand that it will not only affect the patient, but also families and even the caregivers themselves.
Gastrostomy, has more or less immediate therapeutical purposes in patients with head and neck pathologies, such as giving them food support, there are many other causes that can bind to but we are not going to list them in our Chapter. Other times its mission, is to set as a need to save mainly problems or relieve gastric reflux contents, this can determine one of the most significant risks, the aspiration, leading to pneumatic profiles and its consequences, even lethal.
Made this digression, it is understood then that patients with sensory capacities and / or brain damage in more or less degree, we are going to determine that this issue will pass almost unnoticed, from the point of view of these psychosomatic cases the situation must be transferred to the relatives, who are the ones that will understand their needs, no matter how hard it may seem. The installation of the gastrostomy itself, the care tempore and / or the complications that start almost at the moment of the indication of their implementation, care and control of the standard, periods may become indefinite or even permanent. Here, the prescribing physician should give clear explanations of the gastrostomy, to help the family understand that they are capable of helping the patient and accepting it in an understandable and rational way and not dramatize and telling them at the same time about the therapeutic and lifesaving benefits it may have.
Our experience as Head and Neck Surgeons in patients and families, particularly oncological, derived from major trauma nature and or with malformation in the craniofacial area, etc., this means that during the previous explanation of our surgical procedures, they will make out first the therapeutic approach, which our exéresis and / or spotting attitudes are essential and have proven curative intention to proceed immediately to the possibilities of reconstruction. In the case of major trauma and in general, other patients not affected by cancer, there is a component to our advantage and that is that in general, these patients do not fear for their lives, as it happens to the previous, in which the ghost of cancerous disease flies, which is superimposed, usually with mutilating surgery, that will prescribe to them.
It is clear then that once informed of these issues this will help us explain acts more "collateral" as comparatively may be performing a gastrostomy, without major problems in general, considering this act, as less entity, but not something we should underestimate. It is

very common that the patients and their families, which at first are concerned about the risks of the major surgery and the disease itself, they're focusing more on the "less entity, such as the maintenance of tracheotomy, tubes or channels of various kinds and of course, the Gastrostomies, of which they usually inquire whether they still have to carry with it for longer time or when they are going to remove it and they usually claim, will they remove it? ...! etc., and frequently we have to remind them that as we said before, the gastrostomy tube in our case, could be applied by more or less indefinite time. ... And / or forever, but it is not uncommon that they "forget the deal ...."

We have been able, in this rigorous and human reporting, that patients and their families, do not feel cheated at the postoperatively panorama, along our experience we remember of few patients that needed psychiatric or psychological support or even personal assistance or social platforms, thus acting, and to be more precise not even in our radical surgery, with tracks such as avalanches and tracheotomies, etc., permanent or temporary, did we have intolerant attitudes, depression or even autolytic by our patients.

Therefore, we will insist, from the outset, the prescribing specialist, must show the patient and his environment, in addition to his experience and scientific understanding, sincere feelings of the unquestionable need for radical views, but all without going into ambiguities, that may cause ultimately that the patient and his family, will not responsibly accept our advice and search for other options, which may appear less aggressive, such as treatments, chemotherapy and / or radiotherapy, which despite its potential indications and therapeutic capabilities are frequently used as complementary therapy in surgery in head and neck oncology, where they still occupy therefore a less important role in treatment, in the case pointed out, cancer of the oral and maxillofacial region.

Since the introduction and advancement of what we denominate as radical and functional reconstructive microsurgery where dental implants, epithesis and / or facial transplantation have contributed probably in essential aspects in our times of social demand or even social media, to recover these reconstructive actions and functions, such as chewing and even aesthetics, which makes most of the sceptic patients be more collaborating in the decision of surgery to recapture of these capabilities and this allows also the surgeon, sparing no limits of their resections, which is important to ensure with greater certainty, the total eradication of the tumours, as now they are able to expand " with no limits, previously unthinkable or at least questionable" safety margins during surgery, depending on the location and extent of the tumour.

The existence of social support organizations, however, may have and in fact is very important to help our patients and their environment, providing experience, assets and motivation to avoid intolerance and anxiety towards the artificial means of support before us, with the intent to recover positive feelings for the future, and not entering into attitudes of grief or disability and yes for the search of rational and even exciting arguments for the future.

Frequently family members more than the patients themselves are the ones who need help and it is logical that the informed society should get involved in their support, plain and simple collective sense of humanity or proximity, but also practical, since this help, will impact on the patient, which however should be monitored. Although, those directly affected must understand that they will have to strive to seek support and assistance by themselves and not just because they alluded to society may be inadequate, but simply because most of the times they are not correctly informed about their problems or detract from their abilities or possibilities, by indifference and negligent attitudes, so it is not uncommon to institutionalize days of claims for the support and help of patients with certain pathologies.

For all this, the collaboration of associations as in this case, sheltering among other gastrostomized and in collaboration with the Hospital Service Units basically, once they are no longer admitted patients or their independence has increased, should be knowing that they will host different patients suffering from different diseases and that within them, will most likely be situations similar to those affected, whom will understand and cope with the difficulties. Before or at the very moment they occur, or are occurring to other patients. Any medical act is subject to complications, one of the most remarkable for instance, in the case of the gastrostomy, which concerns us is the syndrome called "buried bumper" (internal button gastrostomy buried), which must be considered as a major complication of endoscopic gastrostomy and is not very widespread. Like it is caused by a gastric mucosal ischemia, compression of the buffers that maintain and secure the gastrostomy tube. The clinical problem may pass unnoticed to determine from the output of gastric contents into the abdominal wall surface or even pictures of peritonitis. The diagnosis and treatment, are once again, endoscopic procedures or open surgery.

All this and other considerations in complications should be permanently controlled and are part of good healthcare. We have considered this brief clinical contribution and "out" of psychosomatic purpose of our chapter, which deals with issues related more with "mood", can help come closer to the reality of everyday life, the invasive procedures, and certainly unnatural ectopic, because of its location and type of use, being functional and psychosomatic artificially separated from a multifunctional organ as it is the oral cavity, in conscious patients even for their family and caregivers.

Earlier we talked about the creation of associations for special patients with more or less extreme cases, that are staying home now, or in centres for a more or less prolonged stay, to serve as an explanation of how the care of them and the similarity with other patients who need parenteral nutrition support (AP) more or less "indefinite", which of course, as our gastrostomized, have risks coming from the devices themselves such as rupture of the bag, pellet and pollution content and more local influence, due to the catheter (migration, breakage, occlusion) and / or reservoir. Common being phlebitis and thrombosis and septic complications, medications and even precipitation of air embolism, in addition to those expressed in some parenchyma and major organs like the liver (cholestasis, gallstones, liver fibrosis), and even lipid deposition in the bone bone, as well as allergic complications to latex.

The relationship with family and staff in similar circumstances can be helpful not only for timely care aspects of the procedure but to learn from other more experienced companions, associated with this problem as well, an exchange of emotions, which may be essential for all those involved in such complex environments, but precisely the contact with each others, can fundamentally relieve them.

Parenteral nutrition and gastro-jejunostomy,nowadays, have a therapeutic undisputed or even essential place, and we refer in this case to the parenteral in children with gastrointestinal failure to fulfil the nutritional requirements that otherwise, would lead from dehydration to malnutrition and electrolyte, this can be seen specially in individual cases of short bowel syndrome, of different aetiologies, acquired or congenital recessionals surgery, intestinal volvulus, intestinal atresia, necrotizing enterocolitis, gastroschisis, etc. You can also see, as in diseases such as Hirschsprung disease and idiopathic intestinal pseudo-obstruction where intestinal motility disorders is prevalent, the ectopic techniques we are referring to are unquestionably therapeutic, in sensitive patients such as children and their parents, usually forced to get in an illness environment, incomprehensive to a small, innocent, helpless and so dear being. Very similar to the gastrostomized and the reason why we used it as an example

Psychosomatic manifestations of patients, families and caregivers, etc., may have aspects in common and similar to other patients and their environment, but we should never forget that we must be vigilant and smart, to perceive and solve when possible, the particularities of each case (there are no diseases there are patients, there are no families there are relatives and to be more concrete we should say there aren't medicines but doctors), since success will depend on our therapeutic and partnership with associations (which seems the most ideal) and take advantage of their knowledge and initiatives, they are versatile and collegial, with long and recognized applied experiences and therefore undoubtedly useful for similar cases and the recognition of different and varied individuals, identifying needs, such as hiring psychologists to psychiatrists and even specialized personnel specifically trained, who will cover all the aspects they are recommended for each patient, by the specialists. And as we said, with the main support of the family, along with medical personnel and in this way help the Association, if necessary.

They are highly recommended to identify needs, assessing whether the hospitalization is going to be of long-term treatments, to combat the syndrome that could derive from it, taking in consideration the patient's separation from his beloved ones and their environment, including the social and labour difficulties he will have and those of their families who are taking care of him. Without knowing the exact duration of the ostomy and its possible complications such as the breaking-off of the family unit, disorder of the artificial tract acceptance, travel from their place of residence, reviews, anxieties about the duration of ectopic feeding, disordered eating habits and other open-ended problems, that would make the list endless, it is important that the patient should not bear the weight and the consequences of his illness alone. Even in the best cases when the disease is overcome but the need for a feeding route is still necessary, where we try to minimize the risks it is equally important to keep alert and ready to supply immediate and permanent relief even when everything is going well.

To avoid as far as possible, a greater number of Gastrostomies in patients with oral and maxillofacial pathologies and in general in head and neck or elsewhere area, specially in the case of temporary cases in adults, children, and infants, we have designed our "ectopic digestive tubes" a nouvelle procedure still not very popular which we will briefly describe, but it can help reduce the effects of conventional Gastrostomies in patients with a variety of general pathologies and oral and maxillofacial pathologies often require extraordinary measures for to ensure enteral feeding and aspiration. We report a new method for inserting what we call "ectopic enteral tubes" (EET).

Conventional enteral tubes are inserted into the digestive tract using "ectopic" insertion routes. Currently, the most common routes available are the per cranial or sub mental routes, as well as wounds and trajectories that are present or created expressly for this purpose in the craniofacial area. We report the clinical case of a patient with comminuted fractures of the temporal and left suprazygomatic region, where the EET was inserted.

This new method obviates the need for more aggressive techniques, such as surgical or percutaneous gastrostomy, and the use of natural facial orifices when not practicable or not

indicated while maintaining a viable route for enteral feeding and aspiration. Ectopic entral tubes (EET) is a useful addition to our therapeutic arsenal.
In the world of the face transplanted patients, some of those who are in need of gastrostomy, although our experience is very limited, we wanted them to be as outstanding example to gain a deeper understanding of the global uncertainties that psychosomatic patients, their families and even in some degree medical and professional authors themselves can have, (without taking in consideration the main problem of the potential immune rejection of the transplant itself) through what we call, Organintegration or Pseudoorganintegration, is a term which we will detail in the next chapter, we believe that the patients with head and neck cancer, reconstructed or not, are receivers by default (virtual) and others by the contributions of a new face (real), and this determines probably reactive processes that might be compared to the real transplant patients (effective).
The virtual, the real and the effective, must adapt to new self-perceptions and of others which they're going to affect. You may say that comparing the two situations may not be the best comparison or the more akin to a "simple gastrostomy, but, we dare to qualify what looks like a simple gastrostomy, in some patients with somatic and complex psychological condition, that make the subject with the installed probe match up in personal characteristics of comparative significance with others of the surgical patient's body more ability to relate, this is the face, "mirror of the soul."
The act of feeding by gastrostomy should keep a protocol that is as close as possible to that applicable to a ceremony, relatively speaking, which may correspond to the protocol of a conventional food. Established schedules without stiffness, preparation of the environment (even if most of the time they eat prepared food), meticulous hygiene, availability by the family, etc., in the preparation of the act, with samples of true love and affection for the patient and his environment.
Occupational therapy with training intent mainly, if they were indicated or were possible, for the specific circumstances of the gastrostomized patient can provide even more than those of pure entertainment and therefore may make them feel more useful and therefore more integrated into society.
Dramatically and hopefully understandable by readers, after these sketches psychosomatic disorders in patients with various head and neck pathologies, especially aimed to gastrostomized of this territory, with some notes to other diseases.
I want to take you now as announced, to the world of transplantation of organs and tissues, especially the face, it will be of exceptional because through them, we sense, thoughts and surgical approach, which come from far and by direct contact with them, there are very interesting questions, we want to present, through the new terms, which we denominated above Organintegration and / or better Pseudoorganintegration, with the claim to help understand what that means any changes, psychosomatic structures and conventional functional human being

3. Organintegration or better to say Pseudoorganintegration

We understand by Organintegration or better to say Pseudoorganintegration all phenomena that can happen between the biological transplanted material and the receiver to local an general level, in aspects that range from the immunohistological to psychosomatic and from the beginning we have made things clear, in the present time the referred concept is utopian and incomparable from all points of view, with the one of oseeorientation by some of the pointed reasons and others that can occur, which forces us to specify that the biological transplants at the present time, cannot be considered truly integrated in the receiver,. In transplanted cases with coincident genetic codes and immunological between transplanted and donor, we can be truly speaking, by the moment, of true Organintegration.

Few years have passed since the first face transplant and it seems to us to have been able to perceive, from what the implied professionals transmit, mass media and mainly the observation of some of the few patients who contact generally with the society over some of the capacities achieved from a practical point of view and of social relation, sensorial, functional and even emotional and it is in this sense in where we mainly want to make some observations or considerations.

The direct access to a face transplanted person is for the moment within the exceptional and I would say even "mysterious" for obvious reasons.

Therefore, the material for our considerations, to which we made reference before, we have to understand it from a pure distant observational and with no doubt very subjective, philosophical and even metaphysical point of view, for someone interested in transplants, in this case of face (Without leaving perhaps to point similar details, for external transplants or more peripheral transplants with functional interests and psycho aesthetics, of the central or internal ones, and specially, vitals) as it can be our case, even long before few realized facial surgeries till this moment took place. Where we spoke of our possible contributions of three-dimensional blocks of craniofacial structures for its possible use, in case it happened finally it would be a fact, the subject of the face transplants.

This interest, has allowed us to perhaps appreciate some details that I would like to share with you, with a casuistry so peculiar, for being subjective, distant, dark, scarce, and with no doubt, more likely, little trustworthy from a statistical point of view, and therefore scientific. It is for this reason that our work will necessarily be treated and interpreted by the reader, wisely and even with benevolence, knowing that we have analytical intentions not with critical interest and yes with constructive ones, as it couldn't be in any other way, taking in consideration the exceptional effort of patients (donor and receiver), relatives, professionals and of the society in general, and their representatives, standing before an almost religious fact, highly artisan and surrounded by needs and exceptional scientific means.

The methodological aspect, is going to be as we already pointed earlier, distant subjective and distantly observed, since the means, can be blinded with the particularity of the procedure and not being able to discerniate the scientific spectacle, of the human, the reason why the value of our contributions, must be open critics, without direct experience (it is frequent that some anxious scientists in front of almost unique and uncommon phenomena, dare to give opinions over what they believe to perceive).

At the present time we believe that it is very difficult that a transplanted person of any peripheral organ will be able to transmit his emotions towards that organ and vice versa, feeling sensations that can be considered as similar of those that he had with the "original" organ. It is like the non-existence of the circuit of independence between the transplanted organ and the brain, or we dare to say, between the organ and/ or the transplanted tissue and the soul to make him his in all senses.

I don't want to go further without making notice that the face donor, contributes giving the receiver, through his surgical mediator, a peripheral, more or less complex and always afunctional and morphobilogical cover (pure inert bioorganic material is transplanted, and I call it that way, because in the case of the face and members, they are not organs, in the strict sense of the word, that is used in slang of parenchyma transplants, where they have immediate functional capacities, once connected to the corresponding circulatory system, even being disconnected of the conventional nervous system, not thus, perhaps, of the organic neurotransmitters that can pass on their functions and metabolic influences, through circulatory fluid and perhaps even, of the own atmosphere that surrounds them to the transplanted organ).

It is important to recognize as soon as possible, that the peripheral structure receiver, is the one who is going to give the transplanted material, if it has been done with the best anatomomorphophysiological reconstruction possible, his more primitive functional capacities, very far from the primeval surgery. And I mean primitive functional capacities, because we still have to see, to what point, he recovers functional aspects that reflect more or less clear states of encourage, emotionality, amazement, joy (the eyes of the transplanted person can maybe able to express his sensations and feelings till the transplanted covertures can be animated and vice versa) sadness even a mimic and coherent sensibility with the emotional and psychological situations of the transplanted person.

Without being sceptic, what is transplanted is very difficult to no longer be a "mask" , if it is in the face or an organic prosthesis. These aspects, without doubt, obviously should be deeply commented previously to the receivers so that they won't get a disappointment afterwards which in the future can lead to rejections, not of immunological type but others not less important and very difficult to control, like those that we catalogue like coexistence rejections or emotional dependency between the transplanted material and the receiver, that will be for a life time in the best of cases.

This way the rehabilitation staff and the patient's atmosphere, should try maybe with "tricks" so as the receiver will interiorize as soon as possible the organic and functional sensations coming from the transplant that for an indefinite time will be an inherited biological material, for which a sort of bypass should be made of the most noble sensations of the patient, so that the transplanted person can feel them not from the sensorial and perceptive atmosphere, we refer to sensations like petting, affection, etc for an "organ" maybe little or non-receiving at all unfeeling and really disconnected, or not, in a neuroanatomic sense, but probably neurohormonal and even sensorial disconnected in a central level (fig 1).

So, the nearness to a face transplanted person in an affective or educational way should be probably more beneficial for the transplanted person and for the individual. Accompanied by the facial approach accompanied with the hand shake or giving him a deep and polite hug in the precise moment. Knowing from the beginning probably the transplanted person will have. Activated his sensation of out of the area of the self transplanted, we will evaluate with care the peripheral sensations or any other type that can arise between human beings and the transplanted person others than the ones already mentioned. The way they should look and talk to them in a natural, educated, sincere, sensible, respectful and affable way, without any kind of difference, this is how we will do it with a beloved or admired person for different reasons.

This aspect that we consider fundamental is similar for example when we approach a lady to give her two kisses in a social act, that probably has delicate make- up, prudence will force you to bring your cheeks up to her delicately for obvious reasons and to avoid damaging her make- up. And the habit is to shake her hand she has offered you so that she really feels the affection of the salutation, not through the facial area, which is as we know the area for this social greeting.

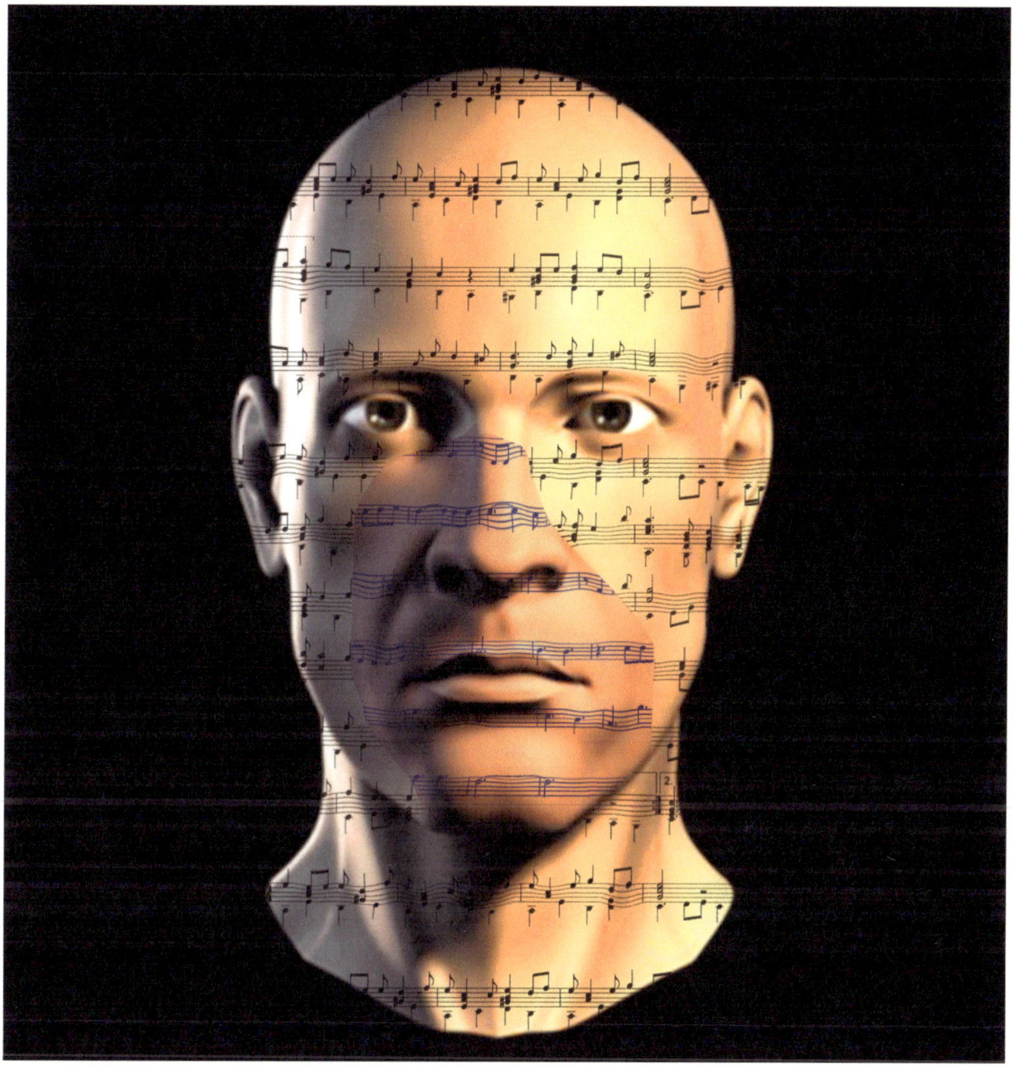

Fig. 1. Musical face
In the transplanted area the music is different from the rest of the face

We should say also that it is not even similar, what a patient can feel when he is submitted to a rehabilitation implantological treatment in the intra-oral structures of the stomatology area with what a transplanted patient of biological material of face or more peripheral areas could feel. In these cases, the implanted teeth have fundamentally functional and aesthetic reasons, but not as demanding and even vital as the one asked for to a face transplanted person which is the individual we are talking about in this chapter.
The concept of integration or Osseo integration of the dental implants, is also a clear example of the organic acceptance, functional and emotional of a biological transplanted person, that we repeat for the first time in organintegration medicine atmospheres, for the moment it is artificial, till it is not necessary to use immunosuppressive for life to try and really integrate it and not in a timeless way.

Definitely, a transplanted organ is not an integrated organ in a biological sense, and we can maybe say, that it will be difficult then to consider it as one in a functional and even physiological point of view.
The human being is the guardian of his physical integrity, and even though nobody wants to have the necessity of an organ transplant, it is not wrong to say that even governments and social organizations should insist in human behaviour in companies,... etc and the obligation and responsibility that each one of us should have with his physical integration, and even psychical, and not to transmit the sensation that nothing happens, that in case of cutting a finger a hand or an arm, you put it in ice and you can saw it once again, it is not that easy, (neither in the case of transplants).
People should be taught how to work and minimize dangers, it is as if our children wouldn't take care not to catch their fingers with the door, etc... something like this, should be done with drivers, workers, ect, and explain to them that their principal obligation when they do risk activities, begins by avoiding injuries and not pretending that politicians are the ones who should take care of us fundamentally. The direct responsible are we ourselves and for that, we have to act in life with all our senses, trying to avoid imprudence that nowadays is more than known to common human beings.
Society has to understand that the best way to avoid transplanting an organ, tissues, is to avoid once again, alcohol, tobacco, drugs and all its consequences, traffic and occupational accidents, all types of aggressions, contagious diseases ...etc, to be more concrete, take care of our physical and psychical health. That compromise is an obligation not only of the governments and society in general but as we just said of each one of us.

4. Conclusions

I am going to finish by saying that when I see an external organ transplanted person, face, members...etc. I first see its aesthetic aspect in global, to look for immediately for fundamental aspects emotional expressiveness and functional, especially in the face. In the peripheric members, we have to priorize, once more, first the aesthetic aspect and immediately next the funcionality, without delaying ourselves looking for more subtle expressive aspects, for example manual ones, that we of course will not discard.
We can't think, in case somebody still doesn't have it clear, that an organ or a tissue transplanted, nowadays, can't be considered an organ integrated structure in a physiological sense, and not only the purely parenchyma (kidneys, liver, lungs, heart, etc) but also the peripherals (face, arms, legs ...ect) as they are constantly submitted to rejection from the receiver, by histoimmunological phenomena and not few times by negative self-criticism supported by the pressure and even well intentioned critics from the patient's social atmosphere.
Note: **Organointegración** and **Pseudoroganointegración** as The Royal Spanish Language Academy, appear new terms, after consulted hundreds of Spanish and Hispanic American Dictionary included the Academic Dictionary (Department of "Spanish daily" Royal Spanish Academy, Wednesday November 3, 2010).

5. References

[1] Pavan M. Patil, BDS, M. Neelkant Warad, MDS, Rajshekhar N. Patil, MDS, and S.M. Kotrashetti, MDS, Cervical pharyngostomy: an alternative approach to enteral

feeding, KLE Institute of Dental Sciences, Rajiv Gandhi University of Health Belgium, India. (Surge Oral Med Oral Pathol Oral Radial Oral Ended 2006, 102:736-40).

[2] Hernández Altemir F.: Letter to the Director of the Great Extra -Very Interesting Magazine- Summer 2002- (Questions and Answers).

[3] Hernández Altemir F.: Sofia Hernández Montero, Susana Hernández Montero, Elena Hernández Montero, Manuel Moros Peña: A versatile route to the midfacial skeleton. *Revista Española de Cirugía Oral y Maxilofacial* 2007, 29, 3 (May-June) 182-187, 2007.

[4] Hernández Altemir F.: Hernández Montero Sofía, Hernández Montero Susana, Hernández Montero Elena, Moros Peña Manuel: -Ectopic enteral tube- Insertion in Patients with Head and Neck and Other Pathologies natural when are impracticable or inadvisable tracts, A new method. *Revista Española de Cirugía Oral y Maxilofacial* (January-February) 41-44. 2008

[5] Hernández Altemir F.: Hernández Montero Sofia, Hernández Montero Susana, Hernández Montero Elena, Clau Terré Fernando, Manuel Moros Peña: The real origen of transfacial Methodology, *Revista Española de Cirugía Oral y Maxilofacial.* Vol. 31.nº.6 (November-December) 367-375, 2009.

[6] Hernández Altemir F.: Hernández Montero Sofia, Hernández Montero Susana, Hernández Montero Elena.: What can happen to the Oral and Maxillofacial Surgery at the Stomatology and Dentistry with perhaps uncontrolled development of the implant therapy or similar and similarly to medicine and its specialties, in matters concerning them each? . *Revista Española de Cirugía Oral y Maxilofacial,* 30, 3 (May-June) 211-213.

[7] Hernández Altemir F.: Information on facial transplantation - "Face Transplant Information) *Revista Española de Cirugía Oral y maxilofacial,* 31.6 (November-December) 403, 2009.

[8] Hernández. Altemir F.: ¡Open Letter to the transplant surgeons! *Maxillofacial News*: No. 38, 23.20

[9] Rioja-Sanz L.A. Doctor in Medicine and Surgery, Professor of Urology at the University of Zaragoza and Chief of Urology at the Hospital University Hospital Miguel Servet, and President of the Teaching Commission. Signe Certificate from the University Hospital Miguel Servet in Zaragoza, which estimates that more ... that Dr. Don Francisco Hernández Altemir, is a creditor of the establishment of the Microsurgery Unit at the Hospital referral ... and also, that early in the eighties, proposed and / or warned of the possibility of facial transplantation with microsurgical techniques in cancer patients with severe mutilation .... Zaragoza on June 7, 2010.

[10] Hernández Altemir F.: Pedicled temporal disarticulation of the upper jaw to cheek (s) as an approach to the regions primarily transfacial retromaxilares and for other indications (maxilopterigoidea Way). A new technique. *Stoma* 1982; 3:75.

[11] Hernández Altemir F.: Pedicled temporal disarticulation of the upper jaw to cheek (s) as an approach to the regions primarily transfacial retromaxilares and for other indications (Maxilopterigoidea Way). A new technique. *Revista Iberoamericana de Cirugía Oral y Maxilofacial* 1983,

[12] Hernández Altemir F.: Transfacial access to the retromaxillary area. *J. Max Fac Surg* 1986.

[13] Hernández Altemir F.: Transfacial access to the retromaxillary area and some technical modifications. *European Association for Maxillo-Facial Surgery, 8th Congress* Monday 15th to Friday 19th, September 1986.

[14] Hernández Altemir F.: Symposium. Dismantling and Reassembly of the Facial Skeleton, Libero Instituto Universitario Carlo Cattaneo. Aula Magna, Castellanza (Varese). Nov. 26, 1994.

[15] Hernández Altemir F.: A new technique of endotracheal intubation (Submental way) *Revista Iberoamericana de Cirugía Oral y Maxilofacial.* 1984; 61:165.

[16] Hernández Altemir F.: The submental route for endotracheal intubation (A new technique). *J Oral Maxillofac Surgery* 1986

[17] Hernández Altemir F.: Hernández Montero Sofia, Hernández Montero Susana, Hernández Montero Elena, Moros Peña Manuel: A versatile route to the midface skeleton. *Revista Española de Cirugía Oral y Maxilofacial* : V. 29. n. 3 Madrid (May-June) 2007.

[18] Hernández Altemir F.: Hernández Montero Sofía, Hernández Montero Susana, Hernández Montero Elena, Moros Peña Manuel: In reference to the Letter to the Editor" A versatile route to the midface skeleton. *Revista Española de Cirugía Oral y Maxilofacial*: V.29. nº.5 Madrid from September to October. 2007

[19] Hernández Altemir F.: Some considerations on the interpretation by the University of Liverpool Transfacial our Methodology and Craniofacial Surgery Pedicle derived therefrom INSTITUTE OF SPAIN, *Proceedings of the Royal Academy of Medicine and Communications Conference Zaragoza*-Volume LXXXIV. Zaragoza 31 December 2004, Pages 1910-1948

[20] Colaborator: Dr. Melendo Julio (Children Gastrostomy) - Head of Paediatric Intensive Cares (Miguel Servet Hospital) Saragossa